BECOMING A NURSE

SECOND EDITION

BECOMING A NURSE

AN EVIDENCE-BASED APPROACH

SECOND EDITION

EDITED BY | MARIA FEDORUK AND ANNE HOFMEYER

OXFORD
UNIVERSITY PRESS

Oxford University Press is a department of the University of Oxford.
It furthers the University's objective of excellence in research,
scholarship, and education by publishing worldwide. Oxford is a registered
trademark of Oxford University Press in the UK and in certain other
countries

Published in Australia by
Oxford University Press
253 Normanby Road, South Melbourne, Victoria 3205, Australia

National Library of Australia Cataloguing-in-Publication data

Fedoruk, Maria, author.
Becoming a nurse: an evidence-based approach / Maria
Fedoruk, Anne Hofmeyer.

2nd edition.

ISBN 978 0 19 558872 9 (paperback)

Includes index.
Nurses—Training of.
Nursing—Study and teaching.
Medical care—Employees—Training of.
Hofmeyer, Anne, author.

610.73

Reproduction and communication for educational purposes

For details of the CAL licence for educational institutions contact:
Copyright Agency Limited
Level 15, 233 Castlereagh Street
Sydney NSW 2000
Telephone: (02) 9394 7600
Facsimile: (02) 9394 7601
Email: info@copyright.com.au

Cover design by Kim Ferguson
Text design by Kim Ferguson
Edited by Amanda Morgan
Typeset by diacriTech, Chennai, India
Proofread by Roz Edmond
Indexed by Mei Yen Chua
Printed by Markono Print Media Pte Ltd, Singapore

Links to third party websites are provided by Oxford in good faith and for information only.
Oxford disclaims any responsibility for the materials contained in any third party website referenced in this work.

Foreword

I am honoured to write the foreword of the second edition of *Becoming a Nurse: An Evidence-based Approach*, edited by Maria Fedoruk and Anne Hofmeyer. This is an important introductory text for nursing students in undergraduate bachelor of nursing programs. The time from being a student at high school, to a student at university, to the role of a nursing professional is most probably one of the most taxing periods in one's career. This textbook offers comprehensive information and guidance to ensure the personal and professional development is incremental, evidence-based and strategic during this intense period for the undergraduate student nurses. During this challenging time, it is essential to foster lifelong learning in resilience and competence in the diversity of skills expected in excellent professional practice.

I believe that this book *Becoming a Nurse: An Evidence-based Approach*, is a timely revision and an enhanced introductory textbook for undergraduate student nurses. It addresses all of the properties of the learning and development experience in life, i.e. awareness; engagement; change and difference; time span; and critical points and events (Meleis et al. 2000). This is done by the advice and information given about nursing practice in the changing work environments. It is impossible to address all elements of development from nursing student to professional in the undergraduate curriculum. However, this book provides critical information on vital topics such as: Australia's health care system, leadership, professional development, career development, expectations in the clinical work environment, evidence-based practice and clinical decision making, cultural diversity in health care, inter-professional practice, teamwork, connecting, and managing safety and quality in health care systems. This book is a valuable introductory resource for undergraduate student nurses.

I truly believe in nurturing undergraduate student nurses and growing our own timber. With the significant challenges we are faced with in daily practice to do more with less, the demands in the work environment, and to continuously renew ourselves through personal and professional development, I expect that this book will be a wonderful evidence-based companion for undergraduate student nurses and will continue to be a practical and relevant text as they become graduate registered nurses. I strongly recommend this book as a most valuable evidence-based resource.

Prof Hester Klopper PhD, MBA, RN, RM, FANSA
President, Sigma That Tau International (2013–15)
Chief Executive Officer of the Forum for University Nursing Deans in South Africa
(FUNDISA)

CONTENTS

Contributors

Dr Lily Dongxia Xiao has a teaching and research interest in the area of gerontological nursing, transcultural nursing, cross-cultural and cross-national studies, nursing workforce development and continuing nursing education. Methodologies she used in research projects include qualitative studies, quantitative studies, critical action research and randomised controlled trial. She won 2013 South Australian Nursing and Midwifery Excellence Award (Research Category). She is a Fellow of Australian College of Nursing, a committee member of Australian Association of Gerontology SA and a member of the editorial board of *Nursing and Health Sciences.*

Dr Maria Fedoruk RN PhD is a Program Director and lecturer in the School of Nursing and Midwifery at the University of South Australia. As a Program Director, Maria is responsible for the provision of academic leadership for the planning, management, development, quality assurance and improvement and growth in the undergraduate nursing program/curriculum. This includes promoting and representing the undergraduate nursing program to internal and external stakeholders as well as developing and maintaining strategic relationships with external stakeholders and communities reflected in Board membership of the James Brown Memorial Trust in South Australia, provider of elite aged care and community services in South Australia. As a Program Director, Maria provides mentoring support to new academic staff and academic counselling to students through the Academic Integrity processes. Before being appointed to the Program director role, Maria developed curricula and taught extensively in the School of Nursing and Midwifery's domestic and international nursing undergraduate and post graduate programs. Her research activities centre around evaluating curricula and supervising higher degree students to completion. Maria has published with students and was an author and co-editor of the first edition of this text book. Prior to her academic appointments, Maria worked in senior and executive management and leadership roles in the acute and community sectors that included a statewide home nursing service. Maria has also worked as a surveyor for the Australian Council on Healthcare Standards for almost twenty years.

Dr Anne Hofmeyer PhD is a Senior Lecturer in the School of Nursing and Midwifery, Faculty of Health Sciences, University of South Australia. She teaches in the undergraduate and postgraduate nursing programs. Her program of research focuses on research education; leadership; knowledge translation; and social capital as a conceptual framework to foster networks of trust, cooperation and teamwork between nurses and other professionals to exchange resources (e.g. knowledge) to enhance quality outcomes and positive work environments. She has diverse disciplinary and interdisciplinary research collaborations in Australia, USA, South Africa, UK and Canada. She has presented at national and international conferences and has numerous publications including book chapters and peer reviewed journal publications. Anne was invited to serve on the Research Scholarship and Advisory Council for The Honor Society of Nursing, Sigma Theta Tau International (STTI), Indianapolis, Indiana for 2013–15. She is a peer reviewer for Australian and international journals and has examined masters and PhD/doctoral theses for Australian and international universities. She has previously served in a range of academic positions including: Program Director: Higher Degrees by Research, School of Nursing and Midwifery, University of South Australia; Associate Professor and Deputy Director, Nursing Research Institute, Australian Catholic University and St Vincent's & Mercy Private Hospital in Melbourne, Australia; Assistant Professor & Assistant Dean, Undergraduate Education, Faculty of Nursing, University of Alberta, Edmonton, Alberta, Canada. She has a broad clinical background and prior to her academic career worked in a range of administration, teaching and clinical environments including community/district nursing, aged care, radiation oncology and over 15 years in palliative and supportive care.

Lucy Hope graduated from the University of South Australia in 2009 after completing the Bachelor of Nursing program. Following graduation and registration Lucy has worked in both the private and public sectors and has had nursing experience within a broad range of specialties including cardiology, orthopaedic and surgical specialties, and oncology. Currently Lucy is employed at the Royal Adelaide Hospital within the Medical Specialties Unit which includes specialties in immunology, infectious diseases, endocrinology and geriatrics. Her current position affords her a leadership role and allows her to coordinate shifts and mentor and preceptor junior staff members and students on the ward. Lucy's career goals include undertaking further study to specialise in Acute Nursing Science and Infection Control.

Dr Angela Kucia is a Senior Lecturer at the University of South Australia and a Clinical Practice Consultant in acute cardiac assessment at the Lyell McEwin Hospital in South Australia. Angela has worked in clinical, academic and research environments for a number of years and was a clinical nurse manager in a coronary care unit for ten years, working closely with student and graduate nurses in the mentor and preceptor role. Angela works with multidisciplinary research teams in the area of cardiology and presents scientific papers at international cardiac society conferences as well as publishing extensively in this area.

Professor Kristine Martin-McDonald is the Executive Academic for the Interprofessional Education Program at Victoria University. She has a long-spanning career as an academic and Registered Nurse. Kristine's innovative vision of an across-institution, education continuum program of interprofessional collaboration, education and practice is being implemented. Students from ten health disciplines move from IP classes, simulations to practice (in a purpose-built IP clinic). Kristine has worked in several universities in Australia and Canada. She has held the positions of: Dean and Head of School, Nursing and Midwifery; Member, Council of Nursing and Midwifery Australia; and, numerous advisory boards and committees across different health disciplines both external and internal to the universities.

Dr Barbara Parker has worked extensively in the clinical environment, specifically in the areas of anaesthetics and recovery and orthopaedic and urological surgical nursing. She has published in the area of obesity and diabetes and has expertise in gastrointestinal and nutritional physiology as well as expertise in programs in obesity, impaired glucose tolerance and diabetes in both pharmacological and lifestyle interventions. Current research interests include clinical skill development and assessment in simulated environments and interprofessional learning. Dr Parker is currently a Program Director in the School of Nursing and Midwifery and teaches within the undergraduate nursing program at the University of South Australia.

Dr Luisa Toffoli is a lecturer in the School of Nursing and Midwifery, University of South Australia and holds a PhD from the University of Sydney.   Her research interests include the use of critical approaches to the issues of the nursing and healthcare workforce, nurse regulation and classification systems for nursing.

Dr Tahereh Ziaian BSc (Hons), MEdPsych, PhD (Health Psych), MAPS, is a senior lecturer and a community health psychologist with a long and extensive engagement in transcultural psychology and public health. The research she conducts offers innovative insights relevant to health services and social support research. Dr Ziaian was appointed for the UniSA's Research Leadership Development Program to provide new leadership for the institution and the wider state and national research effort. She was also appointed by the Governor of South Australia to be a deputy member of Health Performance Council (HPC), to play a key role in advising the Minister for Health on the effectiveness of the health system and health outcomes for South Australians and specific population groups.

Preface

This new revised edition of *Becoming a nurse: An evidence-based approach* has been developed as an introductory textbook for use by undergraduate nursing students throughout their three-year bachelor of nursing program. In this edition, contemporary knowledge and quality research outcomes support the major themes of each chapter.

We welcome four new authors to our writing team: Professor Kristine Martin-McDonald, Dr Luisa Toffoli, Dr Tahereh Ziaian and Dr Lily Dongxia Xiao.

Professor Martin-McDonald wrote the chapter 'Interprofessional Collaboration', a new chapter that introduces the student to the emerging health workforce initiative of interprofessional practice, which is embedded nationally and globally in undergraduate nursing curricula.

Dr Toffoli co-authored the chapter 'Australia's Healthcare System', adding her knowledge of Australia's health care system and how political decisions influence nursing practice using health and nursing workforce data. The authors feel it is important that undergraduate nursing students develop an understanding of how the healthcare system is influenced and operationalised by politicians, bureaucrats and managers.

Doctors Ziaian and Dongxia Xiao co-authored the chapter 'Cultural diversity in health care', presenting an overview of the cultural diversity found in Australia and in Australia's healthcare system and organisations. The chapter also discusses the need for all nurses to develop cultural competencies in their practice.

The chapters on 'Entering clinical settings' and 'Essential competencies for the registered nurse' have been reviewed and reorganised using contemporary sources to best reflect the clinical environments that you as a new graduate will be working in.

The current healthcare system and organisations require nurses to be able to work effectively with information technologies; within legislative and regulatory frameworks; use information to support non-clinical and clinical decision making and be able to translate research knowledge into practice.

Therefore we have included chapters on the legal and ethical responsibilities of the registered nurse, translating research knowledge into practice and health information systems and technologies.

These themes are now new chapters in this introductory textbook and care has been taken to provide you with the relevant information to become an effective registered nurse.

The chapter on 'Safety, quality and the registered nurse' has been rewritten to align with the national changes in safety and quality in health care and in particular the role of the registered nurse in managing quality and safety in health care.

The final chapter, 'Lifelong learning and the registered nurse', reinforces the fact that your learning does not end with graduation but is a lifelong commitment to developing as a professional registered nurse. This chapter also provides you with information on how to manage your career.

We hope that you find this textbook useful throughout your undergraduate nursing program and that it does assist you to develop the knowledge and competencies you need to successfully become a registered nurse.

Acknowledgments

This book could not have been completed without the support of many people.

We would like to extend our gratitude to the wonderfully talented Debra James and Shari Serjeant at Oxford University Press, Australia for their unwavering support, encouragement and belief in this second edition. Their commitment and guidance ensured our success. Sincere thanks also to Amanda Morgan and Natalie Davall for their editorial work.

We are thrilled with the cover of the second edition. Its engaging imagery and colours has an aspirational feel, and portrays the notion of expanding knowledge, deciphering connections that seem unclear, and changing the way we practise. The blurring of colours also brings a sense of connection and drawing together of a series of diverse ideas.

We greatly value the contributions by all the exemplary authors who professionally met tight timelines to make this second edition an exciting reality. We think the second edition of *Becoming a Nurse: An Evidence-based Approach* has been greatly enhanced by the addition of new chapters and contributions by new authors. We are grateful to the authors who wrote a chapter in the first edition and agreed to revise their chapter to align with the aim of this edition, which is to be an introductory text for undergraduate student nurses in bachelor of nursing programs. We were also delighted to welcome new authors to this second edition and extend our heartfelt thanks for their contributions. We sincerely thank each of our colleagues for generously sharing their expertise and research knowledge in their individual scholarly chapters.

We would like to sincerely thank Professor Hester Klopper for writing the aspirational foreword to this book. Professor Klopper is a South African academic and scholar and currently serves as the Chief Executive Officer of the Forum for University Nursing Deans in South Africa (FUNDISA). Prior to that position, she was the Dean of the Faculty of Community and Health Sciences, University of Western Cape, South Africa, where she holds a full professorial appointment. She was elected as President, Sigma That Tau International (STTI) in November 2013 and is the first non-North American to hold this leadership position (2013–15). STTI has over 490 chapters throughout 90 countries. In 2014, she became the University of Washington, School of Nursing's first international Elizabeth Sterling Soule Endowed Lecturer.

The author and the publisher wish to thank the following copyright holders for reproduction of their material.

Australian Commission on Safety and Quality in Health Care (ASQHC) for extracts from National Safety and Quality service standards, Australian Safety and Quality framework for healthcare, Aseptic technique risk management; *Australian Nursing and Midwifery accreditation Council for fig 1.1; Commonwealth of Australia for extracts from* National E-health Strategy. Australian Health Ministers Conference *(2008), National Health & Hospital Reform Commission (2009)* A healthier future for all Australians: *final report June 2009, AGPS Canberra; Flinders University for extract from Student Learning Centre (2012)* Critiquing Research Articles; *Health Workforce Australia for fig 8.2 ; Nurse Education Today for extracts from Caldwell, K, Henshaw, L & Taylor, G (2011)* Developing a framework for critiquing health research: an early evaluation, *and Levett-Jones T, Hoffman K, Dempsey J. et al.* The 'five rights of clinical reasoning: an educational model to enhance nursing students ability to identify and manage clinically 'at risk' patients; *Oxford University Press for extracts from S Duckett & S Willcox (2011)* The Australian health care system, *4th edn; Pearson Education for extract from Sullivan & Garland 2010,* Practical leadership and management in nursing, *6th edn.*

Every effort has been made to trace the original source of copyright material contained in this book. The publisher will be pleased to hear from copyright holders to rectify any errors or omissions.

List of abbreviations and acronyms

ABS	Australian Bureau of Statistics
ACN	Australian College of Nursing
ACSQHC	Australian Commission on Safety and Quality in Health Care
AHMAC	Australian Health Ministers' Advisory Council
AHPRA	Australian Health Practitioner Regulation Agency
AHRQ	Agency for Healthcare Research and Quality
AIHW	Australian Institute of Health and Welfare
AIN	Assistant in Nursing
AMA	Australian Medical Association
ANF	Australian Nursing Federation
ANMAC	Australian Nursing and Midwifery Accreditation Council
ANMF	Australian Nursing and Midwifery Federation
C2	Campbell Collaboration
CALD	Culturally and Linguistically Diverse
CAS	Critical Appraisal Skills
CIHR	Canadian Institute for Health Research
CNS	Clinical Nurse Specialist
CoAG	Council of Australian Governments
CPR	Cardio-Pulmonary Resuscitation
CV	Curriculum Vitae
DARE	Database of Abstracts of Reviews of Effects
DIBP	Department of Immigration and Border Protection
EAP	Employee Assistance Program
EBP	Evidence-Based Practice
ED	Emergency Department
EI	Emotional Intelligence
EN	Enrolled nurse
EPAS	Enterprise Patient Administration System (SA)
GP	General Practitioner
GPA	Grade Point Average
HBV	Hepatitis B
HCV	Hepatitis C
HIV	Human Immunodeficiency Virus
HREC	Human Research Ethics Committee
HWA	Health Workforce Australia
ICN	International Council of Nurses
IPC	Interprofessional collaboration
IPCare	Interprofessional care
IPE	Interprofessional education
IPP	Interprofessional practice
IPW	Interprofessional worker

ISBAR	Identity, Situation, Background, Assessment, Recommendation
JBI	Joanna Briggs Institute
KT	Knowledge Translation
KTP	Knowledge Translation Program
National Law	*Health Practitioner Regulation National Law Act*
NESB	non-English-speaking backgrounds
NHA	National Healthcare Agreement
NHHRC	National Health and Hospitals Reform Commission
NHMRC	National Health and Medical Research Council
NHS	National Health Service (UK)
NHWT	National Health Workforce Taskforce
NICS	National Institute of Clinical Studies
NMBA	Nursing and Midwifery Board of Australia
NQSHSS	National Quality and Safety Health Service Standards
PCA	Personal Care Attendant
PICO/T	Patient or problem; Intervention of interest; Comparison; Outcome/Timeframe
RACP	Royal Australasian College of Physicians
RACS	Royal Australasian College of Surgeons
RN	Registered Nurse
RUDAS	Rowland Universal Dementia Assessment Scale
SMARTTA framework	Specific, Measurable, Achievable, Realistic, Time, Trackable, Agreed framework
SPICE	Setting: Perspective, Intervention, Comparison, Evaluation
SPIDER	Sample, Phenomenon of Interest, Design, Evaluation, Research
SWOT analysis	Strengths, Weaknesses, Opportunities, Threats analysis
TL	Team Leader
TPPP	Transition to Professional Practice Program
VET	Vocational Education and Training
WHO	World Health Organization
WHS	Workplace Health and Safety

Becoming a Nurse

MARIA FEDORUK

LEARNING OBJECTIVES

After reading this chapter, you will be able to:

- discuss the role and function of regulation in relation to professional nursing practice
- understand the nurse's role in the healthcare system
- identify and plan your own professional development
- discuss the concept of professional boundaries and therapeutic relationships.

KEY TERMS

Competency standards
Professional boundaries
Registration standards
Regulation
Standard

Introduction

This chapter introduces you to the beginning processes for becoming a registered nurse. Becoming a registered nurse starts with successfully completing an accredited program of study. All university-based nursing programs must be accredited by the Australian Nursing and Midwifery Accreditation Council (ANMAC).

ANMAC assures the health and safety of the Australian community by ensuring high standards of nursing and midwifery education. Therefore, your program of education will be accredited by a statutory agency established by the Australian government's Nursing and Midwifery Board of Australia (NMBA) under what is known as the 'National Law'. The full title for the National Law is the *Health Practitioner Regulation National Law Act* (the National Law) and was enacted in all states and territories in Australia, on 1 July 2010, except in Western Australia, where it came into being in October 2010 http://www.healthprofessionscouncils.org.au/Reference_Document_Accreditation_under_the_National_LawFINALEDITED.pdf.

ANMAC is also an assessing authority for the Australian Government's Department of Immigration and Border Protection (DIBP), and assesses the qualifications of nurses and midwives who want to migrate to Australia under the General Skilled Migration category (ANMAC 2014).

It is important to understand the regulatory framework that governs your work as a student nurse and your practice as a registered nurse. All the regulatory agencies work together, as shown in figure 1.1 below.

FIGURE 1.1 CO-REGULATORY TOOL

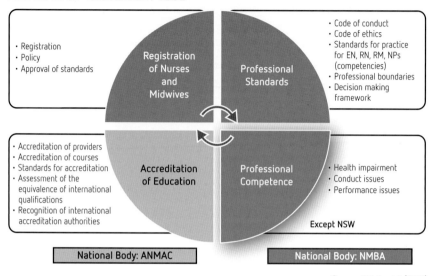

Source: White, J.F (2011)

You as an Individual

People enter nursing for a variety of reasons, ranging from a desire to help others, because a relative was a registered nurse, or because they have been influenced by images of nurses in film and television, or received impressions of what a nurse is from the many books written about nurses. Whatever your reasons, you will bring to the profession of nursing your own values, beliefs about the world and people, knowledge and experience. Your experiences and learning will be unique to you. As with all study, you will find some subjects uninteresting, while others will pique your curiosity and encourage you to explore the subject matter further. Key descriptors for a professional registered nurse include an inquiring mind and the capacity to continue learning beyond the prescribed course materials.

Professional registered nurses also need to be able to develop professional relationships with their patients and with other members of their healthcare teams. You will have already developed professional and social relationships either in previous occupations or in schooling. Before to coming to university you may have been involved with community-based activities, sporting and debating teams, book clubs, or worked with international aid agencies. All of these activities will have developed the leadership, and social and relationship building skills that you will bring to your nursing studies. Indeed, some students continue with such activities while at university.

Over the three years of the nursing course, your studies will cover all aspects of contemporary nursing practice and align theory with practice. The emphasis will be on using research-based evidence to inform your practice. Developing these information literacy competencies should begin with your first days of study. The curriculum which underpins your studies has been accredited by the Australian Nursing and Midwifery Accreditation Council (ANMAC) to ensure your studies are current and meet regulatory **standards**.

The majority of nursing students continue to work while they study, so it is important that you develop a study plan to help you meet your study commitments; that is, assessment, tutorial and workshop preparation. At the end of your studies you will graduate and enter the healthcare sector employment market. Currently, this market is very competitive so, to put yourself in the best position to be a preferred candidate for a Transition to Professional Practice Program (TPPP), you have to ensure that your final grades demonstrate that you have the knowledge and core competencies to be a safe, competent registered nurse. The final grades on your transcript indicate to potential employers your capacity and capability to work in their healthcare organisation safely and competently.

> STANDARD —
> An accepted or approved example of something against which judgments or measurements can be made. A level of quality and/or excellence.

The Historical Development of Nursing

The first nurses in Australia were convicts with no training and limited education. This meant that nursing care as we understand it was non-existent. In the late nineteenth century, Henry Parkes, who is often referred to as the Father of Federation, appealed to Florence Nightingale for trained nurses. In 1864, he was successful in securing the services of Miss Lucy Osborn, a Nightingale-trained nurse who came to Australia with five other trained nurses to work at the Sydney Infirmary and Dispensary (Griffith 1974, amended January 2014).

Early nurse training and education was based on the Nightingale model; hierarchically organised, with nursing students employed by the training hospital. This was the case for most of the twentieth century. Even though nursing was not her chief interest, Florence Nightingale is widely credited as the founder of modern secular nursing. Nightingale based her reforms on the system of voluntary hospitals in England that were already using nurse labour. This enabled her to use existing labour force structures. Nightingale grafted onto the voluntary hospital system these principles:

- all nurses should be trained
- promotion should be dependent on demonstrations of leadership and merit.

Historically, nurses have been defined by the nature of their work and images evoked by the stereotype of the Nightingale nurse (Fedoruk 2000).

Since the 1990s, nurse education has moved into the tertiary sector, and beginning registered nurses enter the profession with a Bachelor's degree. There are now other levels of nurse, such as the enrolled nurse, who may have a diploma and/or certificate, and unregulated workers who have no formal qualifications recognised in Australia by the statutory authorities. While nurses have been in Australia for more than one hundred and fifty years, the regulation of nursing practice began in the early twentieth century. In 1920, the first Nurses Act was proclaimed in South Australia. By 1928 all states had a Nurses Act and the statutory regulation of nursing in Australia began.

Regulation of nurses in 2014 and beyond

Since 2010, the establishment of two national agencies, the Nursing and Midwifery Board of Australia (NMBA) and the Australian Health Practitioner Regulation Agency (AHPRA) saw the beginning of the national approach to regulating nurses and nursing practice in this country. NMBA and AHPRA work closely together to ensure that all registered nurses are safe, competent practitioners. The NMBA and AHPRA have standards that registered nurses must meet in order to continue with their registration. AHPRA has **registration standards** which define the requirements that applicants, registrants or students need to meet to be registered. NMBA (http://www.nursingmidwiferyboard.gov.au/Codes-Guidelines-Statements/Codes-Guidelines.aspx#competencystandards) has **competency standards** organised into domains:

- Professional practice
- Provision and coordination of care
- Collaborative and therapeutic practice.

The NMBA, AHPRA and ANMAC are all statutory bodies endorsed by the federal government under the National Law. All these regulators have been developed to protect the community from unsafe health practitioners, including nurses. It is worth noting that, as student nurses, you are registered with AHPRA under the National Law (http://www.ahpra.gov.au/Registration/Student-Registrations.aspx).

REGISTRATION STANDARDS – Registration standards define the requirements that applicants, registrants or students need to meet in order to be registered.

COMPETENCY STANDARDS – The national competency standards for the registered nurse are the core competency standards by which your performance is assessed to obtain and retain your registration as a registered nurse in Australia.

It is the responsibility of your education provider to ensure your registration, but it is your responsibility to comply with the requirements of this registration. Just as registered nurses can be removed from the register for unprofessional conduct or behaviour, so can student nurses. The URLs provided in this section will take you to the information relating to standards and registration requirements. The National Law states that students must be registered in the interests of protecting the public's safety in much the same way that health practitioners must be registered (AHPRA 2014).

This national approach to **regulation** is closely linked to the national safety and quality initiatives for health services organisations and practices. (See the National Safety and Quality Health Services Standards—NSQHSS (http://www.safetyandquality.gov.au/wp-content/uploads/2011/09/NSQHS-Standards-Sept-2012.pdf).

REGULATION – Rules, guidelines and directives that are enforceable through the appropriate laws.

Critical reflection

Take the time to become familiar with the legislative and regulatory documents provided in this section. Reflect on how you meet these standards at your level of nursing experience. Discuss how these standards shape and will continue to shape your professional practice.

There is a wealth of information in the nursing literature that focuses on nursing competencies from around the world (Chang et al. 2011; Hsu & Hsieh 2013, Meretoja et al. 2014). Core competency standards have been developed to support safe nursing practice in healthcare organisations, and in Australia, these are used to measure individual nurse performance. Grealish (2012) describes core competency standards as the 'preferred technology' for measuring and classifying nurse performance in Australia. This again reflects the national approach to managing safety and quality in the healthcare sector through ensuring that care is provided by assessed competent nurses. This assessment is then the formal performance management review completed annually.

As a professional registered nurse, there will be many benchmarks you will have to reach or work within. These benchmarks include:

- fitness and propriety to practice
- recency of practice
- english language proficiency
- competence
- continuing professional development.

(Wickett & Wickett 2012, p. 102)

MARIA FEDORUK

'Fitness and propriety' (Wickett & Wickett 2012, p.102) refers to your moral and legal fitness as a person; your capacity to work within legislative frameworks and to act with honesty and integrity with patients, families and professional colleagues. The NMBA has a criminal history standard that requires all persons applying for registration to provide a criminal history through a National Police Check. As a student, you are required to have this form of evidence before you go out on clinical placement. Employers will also require you to provide a current National Police Check or its equivalent before offering you a position, for example in the Transition to Professional Practice Program (TPPP).

English language proficiency is an essential competency for all registered nurses, and this is captured in the English language skills registration standard.

Critical reflection

In your study groups, discuss the impact the core competency standards can have on your future professional practice as a registered nurse.

Then, in class, measure your performance against these standards. Can you identify areas for improvement?

The national competency standards for the registered nurse are the core competency standards by which your performance is assessed to obtain and retain your registration as a registered nurse in Australia. As a registered nurse, these core competency standards underpin your practice and create the professional boundaries.

Professional Boundaries

PROFESSIONAL BOUNDARIES – Limits that protect the space between the professional's power and the client's vulnerability.

It is important to understand the significance of **professional boundaries** to all health professionals, especially students. As a student, you may not be aware of this concept of 'professional boundaries'. Professional boundaries in nursing are defined as limits that protect the space between the professional's power and the client's vulnerability; that is, they are the borders that mark the edges between a professional, therapeutic relationship and a non-professional or personal relationship between a nurse and a person in their care (NMBA 2013). Nurses who cross over the professional boundary usually have behaved in an unprofessional or unethical manner. It is important to understand the limits of a professional boundary, especially when you first go out on clinical placement. The professional boundary protects you from being the subject of an investigation when a complaint has been made against you, either by a patient, their family or another staff member. Understand the limits of your practice and always behave in a professional manner.

Professional boundaries may also be breached because a nurse abuses the inherent power imbalance that exists between patients and those providing care. This abuse can range from actual physical abuse to denying care in an appropriate manner, or through exploiting a patient unable to defend or speak for themselves. In such cases you act in an advocacy role for the patient.

All nurses enter into a therapeutic relationship with their patients, using their skills and knowledge to provide care. This knowledge includes information about the patient, which should be kept confidential. The community trusts that nurses will act in the best interest of those in their care and that the nurse will base that care on an assessment of the individual's specific needs. The power imbalance present in a professional relationship can lead to under involvement or over involvement in terms of professional boundaries (NMBA 2013). As a new registered nurse or as a student nurse on placement, it is important to know the limits of your professional boundaries when interacting with patients.

Figure 1.2 shows a schematic representation from the NMBA of professional behaviour.

FIGURE 1.2 A CONTINUUM OF PROFESSIONAL BEHAVIOUR

DISINTERESTED NEGLECTFUL	THERAPEUTIC RELATIONSHIP	BOUNDARY VIOLATIONS
under involvement	zone of helpfulness	over involvement

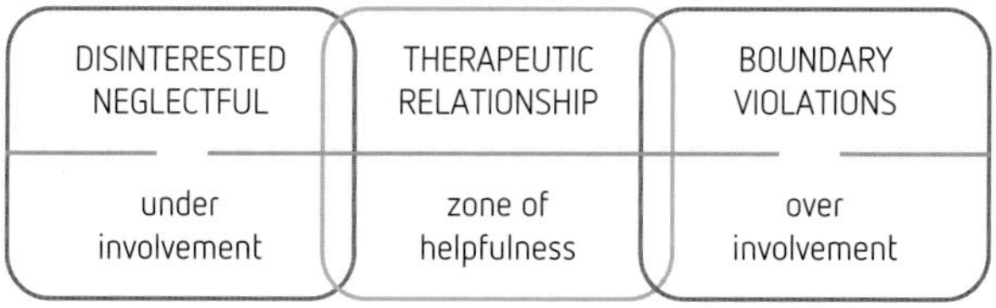

Every nurse–client relationship can be plotted on the continuum of professional behaviour

Adapted from: National Council of State Boards of Nursing (2004)

The zone of helpfulness in the centre of this continuum is where all nurse–patient interactions should occur. Under involvement or over involvement are centres of boundary crossings or violations.

THEORY TO PRACTICE

Mrs X is an elderly resident in the aged care facility at which you work. She has no living relatives. Because of this, you tend to spend extra time with Mrs X so that she is not so lonely. Mrs X considers you her friend as well as her nurse, and you have often done her shopping for her, including buying essentials such as toiletries, and the occasional treat. You have cared for Mrs X for more than five years and she considers you a member of her family. On one of your days off, Mrs X has a cardiac arrest and dies. Some months later, you receive a letter from a solicitor informing you that Mrs X has left you $50,000 in her will.

Discussion Questions

1. Do you accept the money?
2. If you do accept the money, will you be in breach of the NMBA standards and code of conduct?
3. Did you and Mrs X have a therapeutic relationship?
4. How would you deal with this situation?
5. Where on the continuum of professional behaviour do you sit?

SUMMARY

This first chapter discusses your entry into the nursing profession as a student nurse in accredited program of study at a university. You are introduced to the regulatory frameworks governing professional nurses and other health professionals. The regulatory frameworks include the National Law that underpins the NMBA competency and AHPRA registration standards. The relationships between the NMBA competency and AHPRA registration standards and the NSQHSS standards is explained, and so you should be aware that these standards align and shape your practice as a registered nurse.

Discussion questions

1. How much do you know about the regulatory framework for registered nurses?
2. How aware are you of professional boundaries?
3. What are your responsibilities when you observe a colleague's work with patients to be incompetent?
4. What are your responsibilities if you know that a colleague is breaching professional boundaries?

Further Reading

Benton, D, Gonzalez-Jurado, MA, & Beneit-Montesinos, JV 2013, 'A structured policy review of the principles of professional self-regulation', *International Nursing Review*, vol. 60, issue 1, pp. 13–22.

Dixon, K 2013, 'Unethical conduct by the nurse: a critical discourse analysis of nurses tribunal inquiries', *Nursing Ethics*, vol. 20(5), pp. 578–88.

Duffield, CM, Gardner, G, Chang AM, Fry M & Stasa, H 2011, 'National regulation in Australia: a time for standardization in roles and titles', *Collegian*, vol. 18, issue 2, pp. 45–9.

Huby, G, Harris, FM, Powell, AG, Keilman, T, Sheikh A, Williams, S & Pinnock, H 2014, 'Beyond professional boundaries and resources in health services modernization in England and Wales', *Sociology of Health & Illness*, vol. 36, no. 3, pp. 400–15.

Starr, L 2012, 'When is it mandatory to make a report to the NMBA?', *Australian Nursing Journal, ANJ* vol. 20, issue 5, p. 29.

Yanhua, C & Watson, R 'A review of clinical competence', *Nurse Education Today*, vol. 31, pp. 832–6.

Useful websites

Australian Commission on Safety and Quality in Health Care (ACSQHC): http://www.safetyandquality.gov.au/. This website has links that detail the national approach to safety and quality in health care in Australia today.

Australian Nursing and Midwifery Accreditation Council (ANMAC): http://www.anmac.org.au/about-anmac. This website will take you to information about ANMAC and the history of the development of the national accreditation agencies used to regulate nursing practice in Australia.

Australian Health Practitioner Regulation Agency (AHPRA): http://www.ahpra.gov.au/Registration.aspx. This website will take you to the national registering authority for nurses and other health professionals.

National Law: http://www.ahpra.gov.au/About-AHPRA/What-we-do/Legislation.aspx. This website will take you to the Health Practitioner National Law Act 2009 legislation in all states and territories.

Nursing and Midwifery Board of Australia (NMBA): http://www.nursingmidwiferyboard.gov.au/. This website has links to all the information you will need for competency standards, professional boundaries, and codes of conduct that govern professional nursing practice in Australia today.

References

Australian Nursing and Midwifery Accreditation Council: http://www.anmac.org.au/sites/default/files/documents/National_Accreditation_Guidelines.pdf.

Chang, MJ, Chang, Y-J, Kuo, S-H, Yang, Y-H & Chou, F-H 2011. 'Relationships between critical thinking ability and nursing competence in clinical nurses', *Journal of Clinical Nursing*, vol. 20, issue 21–22, pp. 3224–32.

Fedoruk, M 2000, 'The role of the director of nursing in South Australia at the end of the 20th century.' Unpublished PhD thesis. University of South Australia.

Grealish, L 2012, 'How competency standards became the preferred technology for classifying nursing performance in Australia', *Australian Journal of Advanced Nursing*, vol. 30, issue 2, pp. 20–31.

Griffith, J & Osburn, L 1836–1891, *Australian dictionary of biography*, National Centre of Biography, Australian National University, http://adb.anu.edu.au/biography/osburn-lucy-4345/text7054, published in hard copy 1974, accessed online 6 April 2014.

Hsu, LL & Hsieh, S-I 2013, 'Development and psychometric evaluation of competency inventory for nursing students: a learning outcomes perspectives', *Nurse Education Today*, vol. 33, issue 5, pp. 492–497.

Meretoja, R, Numminen, O & Isoaho, H, & Leino-Kilpi, H 2014, 'Nurse competence between three generational cohorts', *International Journal of Nursing Practice* (early view published 1 April 2014) DOS. 10.111.ijn.122297.

National Law: http://www.healthprofessionscouncils.org.au/Reference_Document_Accreditation_under_the_National_LawFINALEDITED.pdf.

Nursing and Midwifery Board of Australia, Registration Standards 2013, http://www.nursingmidwiferyboard.gov.au/Registration-Standards.aspx

Wickett, D & Wickett, A 2012, 'Professional regulation' in M Fedoruk & A Hofmeyer (eds) *Becoming a nurse: transition to practice*, Oxford University Press, South Melbourne, chapter 7.

Transition from Student Nurse to Registered Nurse

2

ANNE HOFMEYER & MARIA FEDORUK

LEARNING OBJECTIVES

After reading this chapter, you will be able to:

- understand the process of transition from student nurse to registered nurse
- discuss the professional responsibilities of the registered nurse in relation to other categories of nurse.

KEY TERMS

Belongingness
Fitting in
Socialisation
Transition

Transition

The *Oxford Australian Dictionary* (2005) defines **transition** as 'the process of changing from one condition, style, etc., to another'. The process of transition from student to registered nurse has been recognised as stressful and emotional for individuals (Duchscher 2009; Rudman & Gustavsson 2011; Kramer et al. 2013a). Kramer (1974) identified this phenomenon of 'reality shock' almost four decades ago in her seminal work 'Reality shock. Why nurses leave nursing'. This phenomenon has been studied over the past four decades because it has implications for the recruitment and retention of registered nurses and, in 2014, when there is a worldwide shortage of registered nurses, reducing the impact of registered nurses leaving the profession and the health care sector is a priority for policy makers, politicians, key stakeholders, communities and healthcare organisation managers (Aiken et al. 2012; Health Workforce Australia (HWA) 2012). In developed countries such as Australia it is becoming increasingly important to maintain a qualified nursing workforce, as demand for health services increases (HWA 2012). There is considerable interest in the nursing literature on the transition process in nursing because of the impact it has on registered nurse retention (Rudman & Gustavsson 2011).

Duchscher (2008, p. 1103) has built on Kramer's (1974) 'reality shock', and, as a result of ten years of research, developed a theory of 'transition shock'.

TRANSITION – The changes that occur over a period of time as individuals change from one state to another.

This theory details how new graduates confront the realities of professional nursing practice within the scope of 'physical, intellectual, emotional, developmental and sociocultural changes' that they encounter in their first days as registered nurses. The four pillars of the transition theory are:

- Physical—the physicality of nursing work in acute care becomes a reality—the realities of shift work; the intellectual demands required of the registered nurse
- Intellectual—the reality shock associated with the incongruences between theory and practice; a lack of awareness of the graduate nurse's responsibilities; the capacity to deal with the responsibilities expected by the healthcare organisation and other nurses
- Emotional—there is often a feeling of helplessness, loss of control; fears of failing, being thought incompetent, loss of identity
- Socio-developmental—little opportunity to adapt to the new role; needing to develop leadership competencies; needing time to grow into the new role.

Transition shock is of interest to researchers and health policy makers at an international level because of its implications for nurse workforce planning. There is evidence to show that registered nurse attrition in the first few months of practice is extremely high in healthcare organisations across the globe and Australia is not immune. (Johnstone, Kanitski & Currie 2007)

(Adapted from Duchscher 2008)

All new graduate nurses experience a level of transition shock in their first year, but developing lifelong skills and resilience to adapt and cope with the transition is necessary for developing your professional identity, clinical excellence, safe and competent practice, and your own personal well-being. Learning resilience and the capacity to adapt is a lifelong process and does not end with your first year as a registered nurse. Registered nurses may work in many different environments throughout their career and will experience varying degrees of transition shock over their working life (Hofmeyer 2012).

In your personal life, you will have faced and dealt with many endings and beginnings but perhaps not reflected on these in any great detail, nor on your capacity to manage these life challenges.

Critical reflection

Reflect on a transition that occurred in your personal life that had a happy ending:

- What happened?
- How did you achieve the happy ending?
- What skills or knowledge did you draw on to get your happy ending?
- Would you have done anything differently?

Now reflect on a transition event that did not end positively.
- What happened?
- What could you have done differently with the benefit of hindsight?
- What did you learn from the experience to prevent a similar outcome from occurring?

Transition to a new role also includes **socialisation** into the new role, developing professional identities and becoming members of new groups. Socialisation involves learning the behaviours, norms and values of a new group in order to gain membership in that group. The need to '**fit in**' and to 'belong' are pervasive human needs, together with developing relationships that will ease the stressors associated with coming into a new environment (Malouf & West 2011).

SOCIALISATION – The process of learning behaviours which are acceptable to members of established groups.

FITTING IN – An important feature of becoming a registered nurse.

FIGURE 2.1 MOVING TOWARD SUCCESSFUL TRANSITION

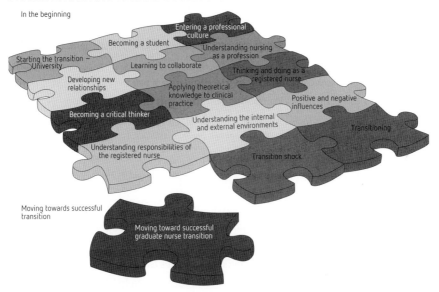

THEORY TO PRACTICE

Emma graduated as a registered nurse three months ago and was allocated to work in the same ward as you about two months ago. Judy was assigned to be a mentor for Emma but complains to anyone who will listen that this mentoring role has added to her workload. Emma avoids Judy as much as possible and asks other registered nurses for information about support to do her job, including you. Some registered nurses are willing to help Emma but a small group of older registered nurses (including Judy) laugh and refuse to answer her questions about clinical care.

You graduated as a registered nurse six months ago, so you understand Emma's plight and need for practical guidance, but you don't have sufficient clinical experience to answer all her questions. You are aware that Emma is becoming increasingly isolated and withdrawn, has made a few clinical errors, eats lunch by herself away from the ward and struggles to complete her patient care on time.

As you leave the ward at the end of a day shift, you see Emma crying on the stairs. She tells you she is overwhelmed with all her problems, so you both go to a quiet place to talk. She explains her current problems to you:

She is thinking of leaving the nursing profession because she is so unhappy.
The current clinical experiences are definitely not what she expected as a university student and she does not know how she will survive coping with the pressure and disappointment.
She also overheard Judy and another older nurse decide not to report a drug error they had made together.

Questions

Discuss how you might draw on ideas from this chapter to:
*   support Emma personally as a new registered nurse
*   advise Emma professionally about how to handle the dilemma in the overheard conversation.

Transition to Professional Practice Program

To facilitate the transition from student nurse to registered nurse, hospitals in Australia offer a transition to professional practice program (TPPP). This was formerly known as the Graduate Nurse Program. Ideally, the TPPP is a consolidation year that enables new registered nurses to become familiar with their roles and responsibilities. The TPPP year is central in helping registered nurses develop a sense of **belongingness**, which helps them move through the four phases of transition. TPPPs are designed to introduce new graduates to the organisation's policies and procedures, as well as to reinforce clinical knowledge and learning.

BELONGINGNESS — The socialisation process an individual goes through to become a member of a new group.

As a new registered nurse, once the initial period of orientation is over you will work as a team member and be responsible for the clinical care of a group of patients. Ideally, you will have received a thorough orientation, as outlined above. However, this does not always happen, due to a shortage of registered nurses. New graduates are often expected to 'hit the ground running' (Greenwood 2000). This means that you may find yourself in charge of shifts—usually after-hours shifts—in the early part of your TPPP. While organisations try to minimise this, staff sick or emergency leave can make it unavoidable. So, one of your learning objectives could revolve around organising staff on a shift.

Box 2.1   A model TPPP orientation

Below is an outline of an ideal orientation program for the TPPP. You will find that orientation programs are specific to each hospital or healthcare organisation, and they vary between each state and territory. Therefore, you need to very clearly identify your objectives and learning requirements.

Day 1
You arrive with other new registered nurses at the hospital or healthcare organisation where you will work. You are greeted by nursing staff from the education or staff development department.

After the administrative formalities (signing contracts etc.) are completed, the formal orientation to the organisation begins. In the orientation, you learn about the policies, procedures and expectations of the employer. You may be asked to express your expectations. For instance, you may be asked 'Why did you choose to come to this hospital/organisation?' Your response is important; remember, the hospital or healthcare organisation is expecting you to be professional in your outlook and behaviour.

Day 2
Further opportunities are provided for you to learn more about your new organisation and place of work. Do not be afraid to ask questions about issues that concern you. This may be daunting, because you are nervous and want to make a good impression, but it is better to clarify issues at the beginning. Remember, there is no such thing as a 'dumb' question. In order to ask the most appropriate questions, you should have done some homework about the TPPP in the hospital or healthcare organisation you are going to work in. The more you find out about the organisation at this stage, the less stressful your first few days on the clinical unit will be.

Day 3
This day may be taken up with assessing your mandatory competencies (as determined by the organisation and, in some states or territories, the registering authority), including:
- medication calculations
- managing intravenous therapies and other clinically related functions
- fire and evacuation procedures
- basic life support or advanced life support training
- occupational health, welfare and safety; for example, organisational policies and procedures, mandatory competencies (manual handling), interprofessional relationships (workplace bullying), maintaining a safe work environment
- managing critical incidents.

You will also have the chance to familiarise yourself with:
- the documentation used in the organisation
- how to manage workloads on a shift
- how to use the nursing information systems to measure workloads and to allocate staff per shift; collect patient activity data, and enter nursing notes
- human resource management processes, such as how to apply for leave
- details such as your leave entitlements, salary and industrial relations.

You should also ask about professional development opportunities that will support and enhance your own professional and career development.

The industrial body representing nursing and nurses will provide you with information. In Australia, the principal industrial agency for nurses is the Australian Nursing Federation (ANF). The relevant registering authority may also make a presentation that covers the role of the Nurses Board in your state or territory. Other professional nursing organisations, such as the Royal College of Nursing, may also provide information about their role and the professional opportunities now open to you as a registered nurse.

Day 4

On this day you go to your clinical unit and meet the clinical nurse consultant or nurse in charge (titles of senior nurses may vary in the different states and territories). You are also introduced to other staff who are part of the multidisciplinary team working in the unit. At this point, you may be introduced to your clinical facilitator, who will be your mentor for the first three months of the program.

Day 5

Day 5 is a supernumerary day in the clinical unit, where you have time to familiarise yourself with the geographical layout of the unit (it is always important to know where equipment, especially emergency equipment, is located) and the policies and procedures that apply to the unit. It is also an opportunity to familiarise yourself with the emergency contact details for the unit and the organisation.

Your clinical facilitator may also provide an orientation program to the clinical unit. This will include the clinical skills, knowledge and competencies you are expected to develop while working in the clinical unit.

You may be asked to develop learning objectives around the clinical skills and competencies you wish to develop or improve while you are working in the unit. You should be familiar with the process of setting objectives, as you will have done this throughout your undergraduate program. The **SMARTTA** framework (Dwyer & Hopwood 2010) can be used to develop effective learning objectives. SMARTTA stands for:

S = Specific
M = Measurable
A = Achievable
R = Realistic
T = Time
T = Trackable
A = Agreed

It is important to set yourself achievable learning objectives that will contribute to your professional development. Your objectives should be achieved during your time in the clinical units.

Remember your clinical facilitator is there to support your socialisation and integration into the clinical unit. While you may feel a little uncomfortable that at first you always seem to be asking questions, this is the only way you will learn. Your clinical facilitator will respect and understand this.

After this five-day period is over, you will be included on the normal roster for the unit. In the first few days of the roster, you may be supernumerary; that is, not included in the staffing establishment. If this is the case, use the time wisely by becoming really familiar with the activities of the clinical unit.

In some organisations, the orientation period continues throughout the TPPP year. New staff meet with their clinical facilitators and the staff development team every three months to discuss the clinical and non-clinical issues graduate nurses have experienced, and to monitor and update clinical skills. These sessions help you resolve issues during your first year of practice as a registered nurse.

Critical reflection

Imagine that you have begun work as a registered nurse. Use the SMARTTA framework to develop some learning objectives for yourself. These could include some specific clinical aspects of nursing practice, and also some non-clinical aspects of your practice, such as organising staff on a shift.

In your study group and with your lecturer, discuss these objectives and how you might evaluate them. What criteria might you consider using?

The TPPP is the formal orientation to the healthcare organisation. Alongside it, there is also an informal process of orientation to the sociocultural norms of the organisation. These norms will be reflected in the culture of individual clinical units, and in the organisational mission and values statements. Once you enter the clinical unit where you will work as a registered nurse, you will be socialised into the culture and norms of that unit. By observing the behaviours and values demonstrated by the people already working in the unit, you will learn 'how we do things here'. You will also hear staff talking in clinical shorthand specific to the clinical speciality. In order to fit into this work group, one of the first things you need to learn is the language of that particular unit. For instance, if you go into an orthopaedics unit, you need to learn the language of orthopaedics, or in a cardiac unit, cardiac language. Learning the language of the clinical unit is the first step in becoming a member of the group. You will already have experienced and observed this in your clinical placements and in your current place of work.

Critical reflection

Reflect on your clinical placement experiences:

- When you went to your first placement area, did you take note of the language being used to describe clinical conditions?
- Did you understand what was being said to you?
- How did understanding or not understanding the language being used affect your ability to plan and deliver nursing care?
- Did you have to ask for clarification of terminology?

SUMMARY

This chapter focused on the process of transition and identified the stages of transition you will go through as you enter the workforce as a registered nurse. You were introduced to the SMARTTA model for developing learning objectives. Using this model during the TPPP will help you navigate the transition process.

Discussion questions

1 What were the critical points in your undergraduate program?

2 What were some highlights and lowlights of your program?

3 How did you deal with these different situations?

4 Did you learn from these experiences?

5 Did you notice a difference in yourself and your approach to nursing between the first clinical placement and the final placement?

6 In a group, discuss the transitions that have already occurred during your undergraduate program:

   i.   your first day as a university nursing student

   ii. receiving the results of your first assignment

   iii. your first clinical placement

   iv. moving from first year to second year to third year

   v.   clinical placements in second year and third year.

   vi. What were the high and low points at these times?

Further Reading

Kramer, M 1974, *Reality shock: Why nurses leave nursing*, CV Mosby Co, Saint Louis.

Kramer, M, Brewer, BB & Maguire, P 2013a, 'Impact of healthy work environments on new graduate nurses' environmental reality shock', *Western Journal of Nursing Research*, vol. 35, no. 3, pp. 348–83.

Kramer, M, Brewer, BB, Halfer, D, Maguire, P et al. 2013b, 'Changing our lens: seeing the chaos of professional practice as complexity', *Journal of Professional Nursing Management*, vol. 21, pp. 690–704.

Levett-Jones, T & Bourgeois, S 2011, *The clinical placement: an essential guide for nursing students*, 2nd edn, Churchill Livingstone/Elsevier Australia, Chatswood NSW.

Useful websites

Transition to Professional Practice Program: http://www.sahealthcareers.com.au/campaign. php?id=67. This website takes you to the career section with SA Health and provides graduate nurses with information about applying for a TPPP in South Australia. Other state and territory departments of health will have similar information available to new graduate nurses.

Australian Health Practitioner Regulation Agency, Graduate Nurse Programs: http://www. ahpra.gov.au/Registration/Graduate-Applications-for-Registration-FAQs/Graduate-Applications-FAQs-NMBA.aspx. This website provides new graduate nurses with general questions about registration.

References

Aiken, L, Sermeus, W, Van den Heede, K et al. 2012, 'Patient safety, satisfaction and quality of hospital care: cross-sectional surveys of nurses and patients in 12 countries in Europe and the United States'. BMJ, 344:e1717

Bridges, W 2004, *Transitions: making sense of life's changes*, Da Capo Press, Cambridge, MA.

Duchscher, JEB 2008, 'A process of becoming: the stages of new nursing graduate professional role transition', *Journal of Continuing Education in Nursing*. vol.39, no.10, pp. 441–50.

Duchscher, JEB 2009, 'Transition shock: the initial stage of role adaptation for newly graduated Registered Nurses', *Journal of Advanced Nursing*, vol. 65, issue 5, pp. 1103–13.

Dwyer, J & Hopwood, N 2010 *Management strategies and skills*, McGraw-Hill, Australia.

Etheridge, SA 2007, 'Learning to think like a nurse: stories from new nurse graduates', *Journal of Continuing Education*, vol. 38, no. 1, pp. 24–30.

Greenwood, J 2000, 'Critique of the graduate nurse: an international perspective', *Nurse Education Today*, vol. 20, pp. 17–23.

Health Workforce Australia 2012. 'Health workforce – 2025', Doctors, Nurses and Midwives vol.1, http://www.hwa.gov.au/sites/uploads/FinalReport_Volume1_FINAL-20120424.pdf, https://www.hwa.gov.au/sites/default/files/HW2025Volume2_FINAL-20120424_0.pdf

Hofmeyer A. 2012, 'Transition as a process for newly qualified nurses', in M Fedoruk & A Hofmeyer (eds). *Becoming a nurse: Transition to practice*, Oxford University Press, Victoria, pp. 35–50.

Johnstone, M-J, Kanitsaki, O, Currie, T 2007, 'The nature and implications of support in Graduate Nurse transition Programs: An Australian Study', *Journal of Professional Nursing*, vol.24, issue 1, pp. 46–53.

Kralik, D, Visenttin, K & van Loon, A 2006, 'Transition: a literature review', *Journal of Advanced Nursing*, vol. 55, no. 3, pp. 320–9.

Malouf, N. West, S. 2011. 'Fitting in: a pervasive new graduate need', *Nurse Education Today*, vol. 31, issue 5, pp. 488–93.

Newton, JM & McKenna, L 2007, 'The transitional journey through the graduate Year: a focus group study', *International Journal of Nursing Studies*, vol. 44(7), pp. 1231–7.

3

Interprofessional Collaboration

KRISTINE MARTIN-MCDONALD

LEARNING OBJECTIVES

After reading this chapter, you will be able to:

- describe the terms 'interprofessional collaboration', 'interprofessional education' and 'interprofessional practice'
- differentiate between what interprofessional is and is not
- relay the global and national context of interprofessional collaboration
- explore the benefits and challenges of interprofessional collaboration
- familiarise yourself with interprofessional capabilities and competencies
- apply the relevance of interprofessional collaboration to the discipline of nursing.

KEY TERMS

Interprofessional collaboration
Interprofessional education
Interprofessional practice

INTERPROFESSIONAL COLLABORATION – 'an interprofessional process for communication and decision-making that enables the separate and shared knowledge and skills of care providers to synergistically influence the client/patient care provided' (Way et al. 2000, p. 3).

INTERPROFESSIONAL EDUCATION – 'IPE occurs when two or more professions learn with, from and about each other to improve collaboration and the quality of care' The Centre for the Advancement of Interprofessional Education (CAIPE 2002).

Introduction

Healthcare has become highly specialised to meet the demands of increasingly complex and, at times, unmet health issues. This has often led to gaps in care provision. As a response to these problems, what has emerged in the landscape of healthcare is **interprofessional collaboration (IPC)** through **interprofessional education (IPE)** and **interprofessional practice (IPP)**. The World Health Organization (2010) has announced the evidential merits of interprofessional healthcare teams as a way to optimise the skills of its members, share case management and provide better health services. The result is a strengthening of the health system, leading to improved patient health outcomes. While IPC, IPE and IPP have been established in many countries for the past three decades, they are still emerging in Australia.

The aim of this chapter is to introduce you to the key concepts of interprofessional collaboration, education and practice in healthcare. You will:

- examine the meaning of terms
- situate the background of IPC development in both the global and national context

- explore the challenges and benefits of IPC
- begin to reflect on what 'being interprofessional' might mean to you in your practice.

Woven throughout this chapter are hypothetical conversations, based on eclectic and accumulative experiences of individuals from different disciplines, to highlight some of the common interprofessional discussions. In addition, there are a number of critical reflections and activities that you are invited to complete.

Terminology and Definitions

Let me introduce you to Jim (a student in social work) and Tina (a student in nursing). They have been paired by their facilitator in an interprofessional unit of study. Neither of them has previously been exposed to IPE or interprofessional content or processes. They have been given their first activity, which is to discuss the terminology and definitions.

The 'language organiser' below is a hand-out provided by the facilitator to Tina's and Jim's class.

INTERPROFESSIONAL PRACTICE – 'IPP occurs when all members of the health service delivery team participate in the team's activities and rely on one another to accomplish common goals and improve health care delivery, thus improving patient's quality experience' (AIPPEN).

Box 3.1   Language organiser

What interprofessional is:
- **Interprofessional education**—'IPE occurs when two or more professions learn with, from and about each other to improve collaboration and the quality of care' The Centre for the Advancement of Interprofessional Education (CAIPE 2002).
- **Interprofessional practice**—'IPP occurs when all members of the health service delivery team participate in the team's activities and rely on one another to accomplish common goals and improve health care delivery, thus improving patient's quality experience' (AIPPEN).
IPP or IPW (interprofessional worker) or IPCare (interprofessional care) are terms that are used to mean the same feature. Various countries tend to favour one or the other of these terms; for example, the United Kingdom prefers IPW, Canada prefers IPC and Australia prefers IPP (Stone 2009).
- **Interprofessional collaboration**— 'an interprofessional process for communication and decision-making that enables the separate and shared knowledge and skills of care providers to synergistically influence the client/patient care provided' (Way et al. 2000, p. 3).
IPC is both patient-centered and team-based, and maximises the strengths and skills of each contributing health and social care worker to increase the quality of patient care (Hoffman et al., 2008).

What interprofessional is not:

- *Interdisciplinary*— 'Interdisciplinary collaboration' was a term used in the 1970s when interprofessional learning was emerging from the evidence that suggested lives were saved with better coordination and collaboration in the health services (Yeager, 2005). 'Interdisciplinary' is a term sometimes used by researchers and practitioners, who analyse, synthesise and harmonise the links between disciplines, to create a coordinated and coherent health delivery system (Choi & Pak, 2006). However, 'interdisciplinary' lacks the inherent depth of collaboration implied by the term 'interprofessional' (AIPPEN).
- *Transdisciplinary*— may be used to describe professional boundary overlap, or health professionals taking on aspects of each other's roles in the absence of the specific health professional. For example, in rural and remote practices which cannot support the full range of health professionals, individuals can be more flexible about their roles and responsibilities. Choi and Pak (2006) describe the concept 'transdisciplinary' as the integration of the natural, social and health sciences in a humanities context, transcending their traditional boundaries.
- *Multidisciplinary*— is used to describe, for example, types of teams or education, and indicates that people from different disciplines are involved in the given activity. It is a term often confused with multiprofessional, despite the clear difference between these two descriptors. Multidisciplinary health professionals represent different health and social care professions—they may work closely with one another, but may not necessarily interact, collaborate or communicate effectively (Atwal & Caldwell, 2006).
- *Multiprofessional*— refers to a number of professional practitioners who work in parallel; each has clear role definitions and specified tasks, and there are hierarchical lines of authority and high levels of professional autonomy within the team. The practitioners consult individually with service users, and use their own goals and treatment plans to deliver a particular service (Griffin, 1996; Ivey et al. 1988). 'Multiprofessional', as a term, may not imply optimal levels of collaboration.

Jim: This is interesting. I wonder why this is called a language organiser? It seems to me to be a list of definitions—boring.

Tina: Yeah. But when I look at it I find it helpful to know what isn't 'interprofessional'. Last week on clinical I heard a group say they were doing IPP, but when I read this, I think they were functioning more as a multiprofessional team.

Jim: OK. There is more to these definitions than I first thought. I like the 'learn with, from and about each other to improve collaboration and the quality of care' in the IPE definition. That makes a lot of sense to me. I didn't know anything about nursing; well, only the usual beliefs that most of the public would have. Having chatted with you I now realise that nursing is much more than I had thought it was. So I suppose I have already learnt something 'from' you, and we are learning 'with' and 'about' each other.

Critical reflection

Reflect on your experiences during your previous clinical learning placements.
- How would you describe the type of teamwork you have witnessed or been included in? Give a rationale for why you believe it is that type of teamwork.
- Why would the facilitator have labelled the hand-out as a 'language organiser'?
- Go back to the definition of IPE. Like many, Jim focused on one part of the definition, the learn 'with, from and about'. Did you notice the second half of that definition; that is, 'to improve collaboration and the quality of care'? Why is this second half of the definition of critical importance?
- Make a list of health disciplines other than nursing that you have been exposed to in practice or in person. Rate your level of understanding of each discipline as: (1) little to no understanding; (2) some understanding but not confident that what I know is accurate; or, (3) a sound understanding because I have worked with that discipline over a lengthy period of time.
- Identify two actions you might take to understand at least one other health discipline better.

Contextualisation of IPC

Tina: Why do you think that IPC was created in the first place?

Jim: Good question. The list of readings might help.

Tina: Yeah, but who has time to read them all?

Jim: Why don't we split up the reading and get together and share what we have learnt. Do you think this might mean we are working collaboratively and interprofessionally?

Tina: (Laughing) Good one Jim. Yes we'll be learning 'from' and 'with' each other.

Without doubt, contemporary healthcare and community services are faced with myriad challenges such as increased complexity of health and welfare needs, rapidly evolving technology, significant demands on health resources, ever-expanding health costs, demographic and community changing profiles, and the necessity of recruiting and retaining a health workforce able to navigate these complexities. These are only a few of the current challenges.

Jim: I noticed in the readings that some have traced the origins of IPE back to the mid 1980s, when The World Health Organization became involved. There are some reports, though, from the early 1900s. So it seems like the idea of health disciplines working together to provide better care has been around for a long time.

Critical reflection

Over the next two weeks take the opportunity to learn *about* another health discipline *from* a health practitioner in that discipline. You may have friends and family who are health practitioners in other disciplines. Ask them: 'What is it that most people do not understand about your discipline?' Reflect on how the responses have expanded your understanding of that discipline. Then, if invited, share *with* that person your understanding about nursing.

Tina: So, it is not a new idea. Look, this article by Solomon (2010) indicates that in 1986 the Ottawa Charter called for IPE to meet changing societal needs. So I wonder why it is happening now?

Jim: Let me read this to you, as Solomon (2010, p. 48) answers your question:

> *Perhaps the biggest shift from the early years is the emphasis on patient safety as a prime motivator. Death, disability and associated costs related to health care error make governments pay attention, particularly when much of the error can be attributed to misunderstanding about the scope of practice of others, delegation of inappropriate tasks, or communication issues. Patient safety may just be the 'tipping point' to ensure that the move toward collaborative practice is here to stay.*

Tina: That does answer my question. Hey, have you seen the *Bristol Report* summary? What happened is quite scary as it 'highlights poor organisation, failure of communication, lack of leadership, paternalism and a "club culture" and a failure to put patients at the centre of care' (Department of Health, 2002, p. 1). It goes on, but it is frightening to know that these failures caused many unnecessary deaths and damage to a number of very young children. This Bristol Inquiry was clearly a turning point in the history of health care in the United Kingdom. How major is that?

Jim: It makes me realise that if it can happen so widely in one country then it can happen elsewhere. So perhaps Solomon is right and that patient safety is the tipping point for IPC, IPE and IPP today. That would mean that in our career interprofessional practice and education are likely to become more evident in Australia. Perhaps our homework should be to meet in 20 years' time to reflect on what we have witnessed about interprofessional collaboration in health.

Critical reflection

Reread the quote from Solomon (2010), as read by Jim above. Now reflect on the following questions:

- To what extent do you believe that IPC, IPE and IPP are now an integral component of contemporary healthcare in Australia, and globally?
- Why?
- What factors might cause a shift away from IPC, IPE and IPP in health?
- What factors might strengthen a focus on IPC in health? How would you describe the type of teamwork you have witnessed or been included in? Give a rationale for why you believe it is that type of teamwork.

You will find the full Solomon (2010) article useful in this reflection.

In response to these challenges, health systems are increasingly emphasising the need for increased levels of well-developed interprofessional and team-based practice. Within the Australian context, the need for an IPP-capable workforce has been identified. No longer is it feasible to deliver healthcare through independent practitioners in order to achieve and improve patient quality, safety and improved outcomes. Some healthcare disciplines within Australia may be debating the benefits of IPC, IPE and IPP (Greenstock et al. 2012). There is, however, a strong swell of opinion from others within those same disciplines, and other disciplines, who unequivocally support the adoption of collaborative approaches (Pieterman et al. 2010). This support stems from the belief that collaborative practice can deliver patients an experience of higher quality service.

Regardless of the uptake of collaborative practice within some of the Australian health disciplines, the direction is clearly set before us, from the Australian health and education policy areas. The following is extracted from a report by the Australian National Health Workforce Planning and Research Collaboration (2011), entitled *Exploring the literature: competency-based education and training and competency-based career frameworks* (pp. 18–20):

> *Within this context, Western health systems worldwide are seeking to define the key criteria and strategies to maximise, promote and support collaborative practice and interprofessional competency. … Effective interprofessional networks offer the potential to identify and resolve systemic barriers to collaboration…*
>
> *At a global level, interprofessional education and interprofessional practice are now seen as being central to health policy … In short the path to the successful implementation of collaborative care involves interprofessional education, which is based on the clear articulation of the competencies that are essential to effective team work and the delivery of collaborative care. Increasingly, competencies are structured within interprofessional frameworks.*

Tina: Ok. My head is spinning a bit now. Can we recap on what we have learnt so far?

Jim: Sure. It seems to me that what we have read and learnt is that IPC, IPE and IPP have been established around to world and shown to make health care systems better which has improved the health and well-being of patients, 'patient outcomes' they called it.

Tina: Yes. Even though IPC is not systematically implemented around Australia, and some disciplines are still debating the benefits, our government clearly sees it as the way forward here. Gee it has been established in some countries for over 30 years, so we are a bit behind in Australia.

Jim: So that brings me to a question: How do we move towards IPC in this country?

Tina: That's easy. Well, not really, but I just read about it in this document (WHO 2010). I'll put it into my own words. So, for Australia to have an IPC workforce in health, there need to be two things in place. One would be what the competencies, and some disciplines call them capabilities, would be. That way we would know what IPC actually looks like in practice. That makes sense. Then the second would be IPE introduced and used in universities and other training areas so we would be prepared, educated and have the experience of IPP before joining the health workforce. So, according to WHO (2010, p. 9), 'a health professional who had learned how to work in an interprofessional team and is competent to do so is an IPP-ready health worker.' So you and I are going to be IPP ready Jim when we graduate!

Critical reflection

1. Read the paragraph below and answer the questions that follow:
'This strong emphasis on building a national health workforce that has well-developed IPP capabilities, in addition to well-developed disciplinary practice capabilities, is increasingly articulated in national and international health workforce policy' (Dunston & Lee 2011, p. 3).
    - What implications might that have on your practice when you are in the Australian workforce as a registered nurse?
    - How can IP competencies build on existing disciplinary knowledge, values, skills, attitudes and judgments?
2. If you are unfamiliar with the National Competency Standards for Registered Nurses, set by the Nursing and Midwifery Board of Australia, it is recommended that you read that document. For the purposes of this chapter, note the section titled 'Collaborative and Therapeutic Practice' which clearly establishes the expectation of collaborative practice by Australian Registered Nurses.

Benefits and Challenges of IPC

Interprofessional practice and education are characterised by strong collaboration between professionals from different disciplines in order to provide the patient or client with the highest level of care or service. Some might say that this benefit is sufficient in its own right to provide a compelling argument for IPP and IPE. However, there needs to be a fuller appreciation, not only of the benefits but also the challenges for IPC in order to address the question, how do we promote interprofessional collaboration in health?

Some of the benefits and challenges are listed here. This is not an exhaustive list but a generalised one. Full consideration would include the specifics of the setting, individuals involved (patients, health practitioners and educators) and policies governing a situation. However, some of the common benefits relate to shared professional experiences and knowledge, enhanced understanding of the roles of other professions, more satisfying learning and work environments, a collective responsibility, better use and availability of resources, shared decision making, team identity, development of coordinated strategies to education and health care to improve efficiencies and higher level communication skills.

Health disciplines each have their own culture; their own professional identity, history and status. So perhaps it is not surprising that healthcare silos and hierarchies have developed, giving rise to a number of challenges. Potential challenges relate to role-blurring, protection of professional 'territory', ineffective communication, development of trust and management of tensions, disagreements and conflicts. Several barriers to implementing IPC are in a relational contrast to the dimensions of IPC itself (Reeves et al. 2011). For example, to obtain a democratic approach and shared decision-making in IPP, the challenge is to address the health profession hierarchy and autocratic decision making. Similarly, in order for team members to value and respect each other, it is necessary to overcome the challenge of moving past any territorial and defensive posturing.

Perhaps the most important process in introducing, expanding or extending IPC, IPE and IPP is that it is done from a balanced understanding, enabled through critical reflection on both the benefits and challenges.

Tina: Ok, this is what the facilitator has given us to do next. Identify the benefits and challenges of IPC. We have discussed some already.

Jim: Let's put it in a table format.

List created by Tina and Jim (adapted from Littlechild & Smith, 2013)

BENEFITS OF IPC	CHALLENGES OF IPC
• Improved efficiency • Better skills mix • Greater levels of responsiveness • More 'holistic' services • Innovation and creativity • Greater likelihood of user-focused practice	• Boundary disputes • Status issues • Language barriers • Competing practice models • Complex accountabilities • Disputed decision-making powers • Imported inequality (e.g. of gender, ethnicity, culture, discipline)

Critical reflection

Disagreements may well be common in interprofessional teams. Reflect on how disagreements can be resolved in a constructive manner leading to positive outcomes for all involved.

Interprofessional Capabilities

It is important to consider what it means to be educated and then practise in an interprofessional manner. To assist with this understanding, it is useful to identify what competencies or capabilities are subscribed to from a global and national perspective. While there is a difference between the definitions of 'competence' and 'capability', this will not be discussed here. Rather, these terms will be used interchangeably, which reflects the way in which they have been labelled by the global developers identified below. The capability/competency domains allow students and practitioners to learn and apply, regardless of their level of skill, or the type of practice setting. In addition, they shape the judgments essential for interprofessional collaboration and are integral to that purpose.

Descriptors of IP capabilities (CIHC 2010, VU 2014)

Interprofessional collaboration (as the goal): A partnership between a team of health providers and a client in a participatory, collaborative and coordinated approach to shared decision making around health and social issues.

Role clarification: Learners/practitioners understand their own role and the roles of those in other professions, and use this knowledge appropriately to establish and meet patient/client/family and community goals.

IP communication: Learners/practitioners must be capable of communicating with a wide range of clients and professional colleagues in a sensitive and professional manner. Collaborative client-centred care demands both excellent two-way communication with clients and excellent two-way communication with other members of the health team.

Team functioning: Learners/practitioners understand the principles of team dynamics and group processes to enable effective interprofessional team collaboration.

Interprofessional conflict resolution: Learners/practitioners actively engage self and others, including the patient/client/family, in dealing effectively with interprofessional conflict.

Critical reflection of interprofessional practice: Learners/practitioners must be capable of critical reflection on their practice and of using this knowledge to improve their practice. Because of its collaborative nature, critical reflection by the interprofessional team collectively is a least as important as reflection by each practitioner on their own contribution.

Tina: I like this next activity. We have to compare what have been identified as competencies or capabilities around the world, including in Australia.

Jim: Actually, it is really interesting that the capabilities are very similar. For me, that means that there really is a cluster of core capabilities for IPC. What do you think?

Tina: I read that there is not a substantive theory of interprofessional collaboration yet. However, it would seem that with this agreement about the core capabilities a theory will be developed in time.

There is substantial confidence to be gained when examining the differing capability frameworks that have been developed around the globe. The similarity across these frameworks is a testimony to what is considered as the core or essential capabilities for IPC. Below is a comparative table of four capability/competency frameworks where domains are identified, albeit with slightly different labels.

DOMAINS	CANADA: NATIONAL IP COMPETENCY FRAMEWORK	UNITED KINGDOM: IP CAPABILITY FRAMEWORK	USA: CORE COMPETENCIES FOR IP COLLABORATIVE PRACTICE	AUSTRALIA: VICTORIA UNIVERSITY (VU) FRAMEWORK FOR IPE IN HEALTH DISCIPLINES
Role Clarification	✓	✓ in 'Knowledge in Practice'	✓	✓
IP Communication	✓	✓ in 'IP Working'	✓	✓
Team Functioning	✓	✓ in 'IP Working'	✓	✓

(Continued)

KRISTINE MARTIN-MCDONALD

DOMAINS	CANADA: NATIONAL IP COMPETENCY FRAMEWORK	UNITED KINGDOM: IP CAPABILITY FRAMEWORK	USA: CORE COMPETENCIES FOR IP COLLABORATIVE PRACTICE	AUSTRALIA: VICTORIA UNIVERSITY (VU) FRAMEWORK FOR IPE IN HEALTH DISCIPLINES
IP Conflict Resolution	✓	✓	✓ in 'IP Communication'	✓
IP Critical Reflection	✓ in 'Team Functioning'	✓	✓ in 'Teams & Teamwork'	✓
Ethical Practice	✓	✓	✓	✓ in conceptual framework
Collaborative Leadership	✓	✓	✓(in 'Teams & Teamwork	✓ in 'IP teamwork'
Pt/Client/ Family Centred Care	✓	✓ in 'Ethical Practice & IP working domains'	✓ in conceptual framework	✓ in conceptual framework

Challenge to Future Health Practitioners

This chapter has introduced you to a general overview on interprofessional collaboration, its importance and critical role in strengthening health systems and health teams with the central goal of improving patient outcomes. It is a challenging but exciting approach to health education and care. Challenging as the erosion of the health silos can inadvertently be threatening to practitioners. Exciting, because working in interprofessional teams does so by grounding itself in the sharing of disciplinary knowing. Sharing this knowledge significantly benefits both the patients and health practitioners.

Tina: Hey, that seems like a win–win situation to me.

Jim: I agree. Thinking in an interprofessional way focuses on the patient as the core business of our work, and strongly connects us to different health practitioners as a team, with fluidness between the team members which is related to the needs of the client. As you said Tina, a win–win situation.

THEORY TO PRACTICE

Case study: The Marsh family's car accident

Mr and Mrs Marsh were driving with their family from a rural town to their home in a major city, after attending the funeral of Mr Marsh's father. The car that Mr Marsh was driving ran off the road and hit a tree while travelling at a 110 kph. At the scene of the accident the paramedics found that Mrs Marsh was 35 weeks' pregnant. Mr Marsh reported feeling 'shaken up and a bit sore in the lower back'. He was also worried about Steven, his 16-year-old son, because Steven 'is a diabetic and I saw him eating stuff at the funeral that he shouldn't have'. The 12-year-old daughter, Kate, was visibly upset and had several superficial wounds to her face and upper arms, and was found sitting holding her mother's hand. After being assessed and treated in the emergency department, the following plan was derived by your interprofessional team:

Mr Marsh and Kate were to be discharged home, but Kate did not want to leave her mother. Mrs Marsh was admitted to the maternity ward as there were concerns for the baby's health. Steven was admitted to a medical ward as his blood glucose levels were unstable and he had hypoglycaemia while in the emergency department.

You are the nurse in this interprofessional team. The other team members are from the following disciplines: paramedicine, social work, midwifery, medicine, psychology and social work.

Discussion Questions

1. Interprofessional team members have different professional roles and identities. Therefore, best practice in interprofessional collaboration is when the team member/s with the specific experience and expertise to best address the patients'/clients' needs take up the leadership role at that time. Leadership has a fluid quality to it. So the leader/s will change according to the changing needs of the patients/clients. Which members in your interprofessional team would be contributing as a lead member/s for Mr Marsh, Mrs Marsh, Steven and Kate? Why? Would this change over time, and if so, how?

2. Interprofessional teams must be capable of excellent communication with each other and with the patient/client. How might this interprofessional team address Kate's desire to stay with her mother?

3. More than one of your interprofessional team is capable of attending to Steven's needs to learn, manage and address the issues arising from his diabetic condition. Who are these team members? How would they best address the overlapping expertise they have on assisting diabetic patients/clients?

4. In your team the psychologist and social worker disagree on how best to assist Steven when he is discharged. How might your team work actively to address this disagreement in a positive and constructive manner resulting in a positive healthcare outcome for Steven?

5. A central activity to interprofessional collaboration is reflection on practice. What are the benefits to the team as a whole if each member is a reflective practitioner?

KRISTINE MARTIN-MCDONALD

SUMMARY

There has been an increasing emphasis on interprofessional collaboration, education and practice in recent years around the globe, especially in Australia. This chapter has invited you to avoid a simplistic or ideal perspective, and weigh the benefits and challenges of interprofessional work, whatever the setting— classroom, online, acute healthcare settings and community health services. It is often the resolution of challenges that raises our consciousness to a higher level, enabling approaches previously not taken. Interprofessionality is a rich field of opportunity for research, scholarship and theory-building.

This chapter directed your attention to the patient, who is central in interprofessional practice, the importance of the core capabilities in order to prepare, equip and support interprofessional students in health and health practitioners.

Discussion questions

1. What is the single most important reason for interprofessional practice in health, in your opinion? There is no right or wrong answer here, but an opportunity to identify for yourself what that might be.

2. Identify an experience where you or a family member has had healthcare or community service delivered by more than one type of healthcare practitioner. What interprofessional capabilities were evident, or in what ways might the interprofessional collaboration have been improved?

3. The discipline of nursing has one, if not the highest number, of practitioners. What, if any, responsibilities might this mean for nurses to ensure they collaborate in an interprofessional manner?

4. The development and sustainability of an interprofessional culture in health requires support at the organisational level. Describe one support strategy for each of the following organisations that might be achieved: (a) Professional association (b) Discipline accreditation body and (c) Healthcare service.

5. Respect for one another as individuals must be paralleled by respect for each other's professional identity and practice. Discuss why this is a critical principle for interprofessional collaboration.

Further Reading

Interprofessional education resources

Bainbridge, LA 2009, *The power of prepositions: learning with, from, and about others in interprofessional health education*, Union Institute & University, Cincinnati, Ohio.

Freeth, D, Hammick, M, Reeves, S, Koppel, I & Barr, H 2005, *Effective interprofessional education: development, delivery and evaluation*. Blackwell Publishing Ltd, CAIPE.

Howkins, E. & Bray, J (eds) 2008, *Preparing interprofessional teaching: theory and practice*, Radcliffe Publishing, Oxford.

Interprofessional practice resources

Dean, SG, Siegert, RJ & Taylor, WJ (eds) 2012, *Interprofessional rehabilitation: a person-centred approach*, Wiley-Blackwell, Oxford.

Pollard, KC, Thomas, J & Miers, M (eds) 2010, *Understanding interprofessional working in health and social care*, Palgrave Macmillan, New York.

Trod, L & Chivers, L (eds) 2011, *Interprofessional working in practice: learning and working together for children and families*, Open University Press, Berkshire.

Interprofessional collaboration resources

Bromage, A, Clouder, L, Thistlethwaite, J & Gordon, F 2010, *Interprofessional e-learning and collaborative work: practices and technologies*, Information Science Reference, New York.

Reeves, S, Lewin, S, Espin, S & Zwarenstein, M 2010, *Interprofessional teamwork for health and social care*, Wiley-Blackwell, Oxford.

Royeen, CB, Jensen, GM & Harvan, RA 2009, *Leadership in interprofessional health education and practice*, Jones and Bartlett publishers, Massachusetts.

Useful websites

A Framework for Interprofessional Education in the Health Disciplines (Victoria University, Australia), Interprofessional Education Program: www.vu.edu.au/interprofessional-education-program-ipep.

Australasian Interprofessional Practice & education Network (AIPPEN) http://www.aippen.net/

Canadian Interprofessional Health Collaborative (CIHC) and Competency Framework: http://www.cihc.ca/ and http://www.cihc.ca/files/CIHC_IPCompetencies_Feb1210.pdf.

Centre for the Advancement of Interprofessional Education CAIPE: http://caipe.org.uk/

Core Competencies for Interprofessional Collaborative Practice (USA): www.aacn.nche.edu/education-resources/ipecreport.pdf.

Interprofessional Capability Framework: A framework containing capabilities and learning levels leading to interprofessional capability (UK): www.cuilu.group.shef.ac.uk/capability_framework.pdf.

References

Atwal, A, & Caldwell, K 2006, 'Nurses' perceptions of multidisciplinary team work in acute health-care', *International Journal of Nursing Practice*, vol. 12(6), pp. 359–60.

Australian National Health Workforce Planning and Research Collaboration 2011, *Exploring the literature: competency-based education and training and competency-based career frameworks*, The University of Queensland, Australia.

Australasian Interprofessional Education and Practice Association, accessed 11 September, 2012, http://www.aippen.net.

Centre for the Advancement of Interprofessional Education (CAIPE) 2002 *Defining IPE*, accessed 8 September 2013, http://www.caipe.org.uk/about-us/defining-ipe

Choi, BC, & Pak, AW 2006, 'Multidisciplinarity, interdisciplinarity and transdisciplinarity in health research, services, education and policy: 1. Definitions, objectives, and evidence of effectiveness', *Clinical Investigative Medicine*, vol. 29(6), pp. 351–64.

Department of Health, UK 2002, 'Learning from Bristol: The DH response to the report of the public inquiry into children's heart surgery at the Bristol Royal Infirmary 1984–1995', accessed 8 January 2014 from DH UK archives: http://webarchive. nationalarchives.gov.uk/20130107105354/http://www.dh.gov.uk/prod_consum_dh/ groups/dh_digitalassets/@dh/@en/documents/digitalasset/dh_4082232.pdf.

Dunston, R & Lee, A 2011, *Curriculum renewal for interprofessional education in health*, University of Technology, Sydney.

Greenstock, LN, Brooks, PM, Webb, GR, & Moran, MC 2012, 'Taking stock of interprofessional learning in Australia', *Medical Journal of Australia*, vol. 196(11), pp. 1–4.

Griffin, S 1996, 'Occupational therapists as health care team members: a review of the literature', *Australian Occupational Therapy Journal*, vol. 43(1), pp. 83–94.

Hoffman, SJ, Rosenfield, D, Gilbert, JHV & Oandasan, IF 2008, 'Student leadership in interprofessional education: benefits, challenges and implications for educators, researchers and policymakers', *Medical Education*, vol. 42(7), pp. 654–61.

Ivey, SL, Brown, KS, Teske, Y & Silverman, D 1988, 'About interdisciplinary practice in health care settings', *Journal of Allied Health*, vol. 17, pp. 189–95.

Littlechild, B & Smith, R 2013, *A handbook for interprofessional practice in the human services*. Pearson Education Ltd, Essex.

Pieterman, L, Newton, JM & Canny, BJ 2010, 'Interprofessional education for interprofessional practice: does it make a difference?', *Medical Journal of Australia*, vol. 193(2), pp. 92–3.

Reeves, S, Lewin, S, Espin, S & Swarenstein, M 2011, *Interprofessional teamwork for health and social care*, Oxford: Wiley-Blackwell.

Solomon, P 2010 'Inter-professional collaboration: passing fad or way of the future?', *Physiotherapy Canada*, vol. 62(1), pp. 47–55.

Stone, J 2009, *IPCP: Definitions and terminology*, ACT Health Service, Australia.

Way, D, Jones, L & Busing, N 2000, 'Implementing strategies: collaboration in primary care— family doctors & nurse practitioners delivering shared care', Discussion paper written for the Ontario College of Family Physicians.

World Health Organization 2010, 'framework for action on interprofessional education and collaborative practice', accessed from the World Health Organization: http://www. who.int/hrh/nursing_midwifery/en/

Yeager, S 2005, 'Interdisciplinary collaboration: the heart and soul of health care', *Critical Care Nursing Clinics of North America*, vol. 17(2).

Cultural Diversity in Healthcare

TAHEREH ZIAIAN AND LILY DONGXIA XIAO

LEARNING OBJECTIVES

After reading this chapter, you will be able to:

- describe the cultural and linguistic characteristics of Australia's population
- define and explain 'cultural competence' in the Australian cultural context
- define and explain 'cultural competency' in cross-cultural communication
- discuss how to achieve culturally and linguistically appropriate care in patient–nurse cross-cultural interactions
- discuss how to achieve cultural competency in nurse–nurse cross-cultural interactions
- identify useful information and resources to support culturally and linguistically appropriate care for patients
- describe the process best suited to promoting quality care and cultural safety specifically for patients and their families from diverse racial, ethno-cultural and language backgrounds
- define and examine strategies for promoting effective cross-cultural communication in the multicultural workplace.

KEY TERMS

Cross-cultural communication
Culturally and linguistically diverse background (CALD)
Culture
Transcultural nursing

Cultural Diversity in Australia

Australia possesses one of the most diverse populations in the world, evidenced by its Aboriginal and Torres Strait Islander peoples, and people who have arrived here from all over the world through various immigration and humanitarian programs. These diverse populations also make Australia the most culturally diverse nation in the world. **Culture** is defined as 'a learned, patterned behavioural response acquired over time that includes implicit versus explicit beliefs, attitudes, values, customs, norms, taboos, arts, and lifeways accepted by a community of individuals' (Purnell 2011, p. 528). This definition acknowledges the impact that ethnicity, religion, spirituality and other factors have on the formation of culture. It also suggests that culture held by individuals and groups of people is not static, but changes over

CULTURE – A learned, patterned behavioural response acquired over time that includes implicit and explicit beliefs, attitudes, values, customs, norms, taboos, arts, and lifeways accepted by a community of individuals.

time, influenced by social and environmental factors. This is particularly true for many immigrants, who have changed their culture from the country of origin and adapted to Australian culture (Purnell 2011).

As a nurse, you need to be aware that making assumptions about a patient's culture prior to nursing assessment may be associated with stereotyping. Such attitudes towards patients not only negatively impact on nurse–patient therapeutic relationships, but also contribute to unmet care needs for the patient.

As a nation built on immigration, diversity in Australia is related to linguistic, religious and cultural diversity. People in Australia come from over 200 different countries, practice over 116 religions (Johnstone and Kanitsaki 2005), and speak over 260 languages (Department of Immigration and Citizenship 2011). In the 2011 census, 80 per cent of the Australian population aged five and over reported that they only spoke English at home, while 2 per cent did not speak English at all. English proficiency varied among populations who indicated that English was not their first language (Australian Bureau of Statistics 2012). It is officially acknowledged that Australia is not only a 'multicultural society' (Commonwealth of Australia 1999), but also one of the most culturally and linguistically diverse societies in the world. Such diversity requires constructive relationships and interactions between members of these various groups. Culturally and linguistically diverse patient populations pose communication challenges in nurse–patient cross-cultural interactions. There is a high possibility that a nurse may misunderstand and misinterpret meanings from a patient who cannot speak English well or is unable to speak it at all. Patient safety and quality of care can be threatened in such situations. Healthcare organisations usually have policies and procedures to guide cross-cultural communication. You will need to be familiar with and act according to these policies and procedures in every organisation in which you work throughout your career as a registered nurse.

CULTURALLY AND LINGUISTICALLY DIVERSE (CALD) BACKGROUND— A person who differs from the mainstream culture according to religion and spirituality, racial background and ethnicity, as well as language.

The term **culturally and linguistically diverse (CALD) background** has been widely used in the Australian Government's reports, and refers to the range of groups that differ in culture and language in the Australian population (NHMRC 2006). Based on the 2011 census, 46 per cent of Australians were either born overseas or have a parent who was born overseas (Australian Bureau of Statistics 2012). The countries representing the highest overseas-born populations in 2011 are the United Kingdom (19.6 per cent), New Zealand (7.4 per cent), the People's Republic of China (6.5 per cent), India (5.7 per cent) and Vietnam (3.5 per cent) (Department of Immigration and Citizenship 2013). The most common languages spoken at home, other than English, were Mandarin (1.7 per cent), Italian (1.5 per cent), Arabic (1.4 per cent), Cantonese (1.3 per cent) and Greek (1.3 per cent) in 2011.

Culture and English proficiency impact on an individual's health in Australia in various ways. First, culture-associated values, beliefs and behaviours may be protectors or risk factors of a disease. Therefore, the prevalence and incidence of a disease may vary among different cultural groups. For example, studies have shown that incidence of lung cancer is higher among female migrants from the United Kingdom, but lower in female migrants from Asian countries, due to differences in smoking rates (NHMRC 2006). Second, cultural beliefs about certain diseases may also contribute to the delay in seeking medical diagnosis and treatment. For example, some cultural groups view dementia as part of normal ageing and believe medical treatment is not helpful (Alzheimers' Australia 2011). Third, people from CALD backgrounds face more challenges to access and use healthcare services or resources because of a lack of social networks, language barriers, and a lack of culturally and linguistically appropriate services and resources (NHMRC 2006). As a nurse, you need to be knowledgeable about factors affecting the health of the groups you serve in order to improve the health of all.

Multicultural nursing workforce

The Australian nursing workforce has also become increasingly multicultural in the past decade, partially because of the use of immigrant nurses to fill nursing vacancies (AIHW 2009). Based on recent information, overseas-qualified nurses have constituted approximately 15.5 per cent of the nursing population (AIHW 2009). The donor countries of these nurses have shifted from mainly English-speaking nations to non-English-speaking nations (AIHW 2009). Fifty-six per cent of nursing students were born overseas, and international nursing students make up approximately 18 per cent of the nursing student population (Jeong et al. 2011; Salamonson et al. 2012). The diversity of the nursing workforce has implications for care delivery in clinical settings and for the integration of immigrant nurses into the mainstream nursing workforce.

It has been recognised that a healthcare workforce that reflects Australia's diverse population is a strength in delivering culturally and linguistically appropriate healthcare, and reduces healthcare disparity in a multicultural society (NHMRC 2006; Office of Minority Health 2013). Actively recruiting healthcare workers from CALD backgrounds to provide ethno-specific healthcare services has been used as a strategy to improve healthcare for CALD groups in Australia (NHMRC 2006; Department of Health and Ageing 2012). The growing diversity of nurses and other professionals in the healthcare system frequently poses challenges as well as opportunities in the multicultural team setting. Studies have shown that multicultural teams have advantages in that they better generate new ideas and solutions to meet care needs for patients and clients from CALD backgrounds (Dreachslin et al. 2000). In addition, team members are able to act as cultural brokers to address patients' care needs (Xiao et al. 2013). However, multicultural teams are also associated with disadvantages, such as the difficulty of communicating and collaborating among team members from diverse backgrounds (Dreachslin et al. 2000; Xiao et al. 2013). The way to improve teamwork is to develop cultural competence and learn from each other's culture and communication style.

Culturally Competent Care—What is it?

Culturally competent healthcare is built on the principle that 'all Australasians should be able to access government programs and services equitably, regardless of their cultural or linguistic backgrounds' (Department of Immigration and Citizenship 2013). The primary goal of culturally competent care is to ensure the provision of quality care in a safe environment to people of diverse racial, language and ethno-specific cultural backgrounds; to minimise the disparities in healthcare that these minority groups suffer compared to the mainstream population (Johnston & Kanitsaki 2005). A cultural competency model in healthcare has been studied by the National Health and Medical Research Council (NHMRC) in Australia in the context of health promotion and can be used as a guide for nursing practice. Cultural competency standards in the model are organised in four dimensions, including healthcare system, healthcare organisations, healthcare professions and individual health professionals. Culture competency is defined by the NHMRC as:

> Cultural competency is a set of congruent behaviours, attitudes, and policies that come together in a system, agency or among professionals and enable that system, agency or those professionals to work effectively in cross-cultural situations (Cross et al. 1989, p. 7). Cultural competency is much more than awareness of cultural differences, as it focuses on the capacity of the health system to improve health and wellbeing by integrating culture into the delivery of health services (NHMRC 2006, p. 7).

This definition, along with the four-dimension cultural competency standards, emphasises the capacity of the healthcare system, taking into account people's cultural beliefs, behaviours and needs. It considers that cultural competence is a process as well as an output, synthesising both knowledge and skills obtained during the personal and professional life of individuals (Papadopoulos 2006). This systematic approach is necessary to tackle problems such as stereotyping, prejudiced attitudes, mistreatment, and discrimination towards patients or co-workers in the multicultural environment. Developing cultural competency in health care requires sustained solutions through policy changes, resource development and education programs. This definition also emphasises the change of practice for improved care outcomes for patients through the development of cultural competency in the healthcare system. Information on cultural competency in Australia's healthcare system is available from the National Health and Medical Research Council (NHMRC) online at http://www.nhmrc.gov.au/_files_nhmrc/publications/attachments/hp19.pdf.

The nursing profession has committed itself to cultural competence. Australia has a remarkable consciousness which recognises and values cultural diversity and sees diversity as a strength rather than a weakness. In fact, in Australia, cultural diversity is viewed as an integral part of the social system. At the professional practice level, cultural competency for registered nurses has been integrated into the national competency standards for the registered nurse across the four domains of professional practice, comprising critical thinking, provision and coordination of care, and collaborative and therapeutic practice (Nursing and Midwifery Board of Australia 2010). These are available on the Nursing and Midwifery Board of Australia (NMBA) website online at: http://www.nursingmidwiferyboard.gov.au/Codes-Guidelines-Statements/Codes-Guidelines.aspx.

The cultural competency standards cover the attitudes, knowledge and skills that are necessary when delivering culturally and linguistically appropriate care to patients. You need to be familiar with these standards and demonstrate that you have met them in care settings.

Transcultural nursing

Cultural competency in nursing practice has been heavily researched in the past four decades in the United States of America, led by Dr Madeleine Leininger, (13 July 1925–10 August 2012) (Transcultural Nursing Society 2012). Dr Leininger was the founder of transcultural nursing and established the Transcultural Nursing Society in 1974. She commenced her transcultural nursing journey in the 1960s and contributed to the development of transcultural nursing theory, nursing education and practice to improve cultural competency in healthcare. Today, many universities in the United States offer transcultural education for nurses and prepare them to be licensed transcultural nursing specialists (Transcultural Nursing Society 2012). Information on the Transcultural Nursing Society and resources it provides is available online at http://www.tcns.org/index.html, or search 'Transcultural Nursing Society'.

Transcultural nursing is defined as a field of nursing in which the nurse interacts with patients in intercultural encounters, identifies care needs and

TRANSCULTURAL NURSING – A field of nursing in which the nurse interacts with clients in intercultural encounters, identifies care needs and delivers care that is culturally congruent for the clients.

delivers care that is culturally congruent and safe for the patients (Leininger 2006). Leininger's 'Cultural Care Diversity and Universality' (or Cultural Care Theory) is based on the major assumptions listed below (Leininger 2006, pp. 18–19):

- Caring is essential to curing and healing.
- Every human culture has generic, folk, or indigenous care knowledge and practices.
- Cultural care values, beliefs and practices are influenced by, and tend to be embedded in the worldview, language, philosophy, religion, spirituality, kinship, social, political, legal, educational, economic, technological, ethno-historical, and environmental context.

Leininger's Cultural Care Theory is illustrated in her 'Sunrise Enabler to Discover Cultural Care' Model and is frequently cited in transcultural education and research programs. It illustrates the existence of folk care–cure practices in every culture and how to approach patients' folk care–cure practice in order to achieve culturally congruent care and optimise care outcomes. However, Leininger's Sunrise Model has been viewed as lacking practical approaches to help nurses assess patients' care needs in clinical settings (Giger 2013). Moreover, the nurse is in a dominant position to determine the culturally congruent care, and this may be associated with cultural bias or stereotyping in the absence of critical reflection (Campesino 2008). In addition, transcultural nursing theory has also been criticised as overlooking power imbalances between the majority group and the minority group and social structures (policies and resources) that contribute to the health disparities among cultural groups in a multicultural society (Campesino 2008). As a nurse, you need to be aware of these factors as they affect the healthcare of patients from CALD backgrounds, and demonstrate the ability to advocate on behalf of patients and their communities.

Cultural safety

Cultural safety was originally developed in New Zealand more than two decades ago to respond to the concerns about unmet care needs of the Maori people (Nursing Council of New Zealand 2011). This concept of cultural competency emphasises the care recipient's perspective as to whether care services are culturally appropriate. Cultural safety has been evolved to address culturally competent care in cross-cultural encounters. The Nursing Council of New Zealand (2011, p. 7) defines 'cultural safety' as:

> *The effective nursing practice of a person or family from another culture, and is determined by that person or family. Culture includes, but is not restricted to, age or generation; gender; sexual orientation; occupation and socioeconomic status; ethnic origin or migrant experience; religious or spiritual belief; and disability.*

The nurse delivering the nursing service will have undertaken a process of reflection on his or her own cultural identity and will recognise the impact that his or her personal culture has on his or her professional practice. Unsafe cultural practice comprises any action which diminishes, demeans or disempowers the cultural identity and well-being of an individual.

The definition points out that cultural safety can only be achieved through the nurse's critical reflection as to the impact of his or her own culture, and the relations of power between the nurse and the patient on culturally appropriate care. This approach to developing nurses' cultural competency attempts to overcome some of the weaknesses identified in transcultural nursing. In addition, the component of critical reflection embedded in cultural safety is also suitable for the cross-cultural situation, where a nurse from an immigrant background delivers care to a patient from the majority through the patient's perspectives of culturally appropriate care.

Critical reflection

In your study group, reflect on the cross-cultural interactions you may have had with patients during your clinical placements.
- Discuss what strategies you will use to empower patients or their families to participate in planning, implementing and evaluating nursing care in cross-cultural situations.
- Besides transcultural nursing and cultural safety, there are many other theories and models being developed to address culturally competent care for patients. Discuss how you will update your knowledge in cross-cultural care through a lifelong learning pathway. Which databases and information sources do you usually access to update your nursing knowledge in cross-cultural care?

Cultural competency in cross-cultural communication

Competent **cross-cultural communication** is a crucial part of cultural competency in health care. 'Cross-cultural communication' is defined as 'the symbolic exchange process whereby individuals from two (or more) different cultural communities negotiate shared meanings in an interactive situation' (Ting-Toomey 1999, p. 16). Studies have identified that people from the same cultural background share some patterns of thinking and behaviours in communication. In order to simplify these patterns, cultures are grouped into individualist culture and collectivist culture (Ting-Toomey 2010). However, no one culture is purely individualistic or collectivist, but most cultures will have a tendency towards one or the other.

CROSS-CULTURAL COMMUNICATION—
A symbolic exchange process whereby individuals from two (or more) different cultural communities negotiate shared meanings in an interactive situation.

Individualist cultures versus collectivist cultures

Individualist cultures encourage individualist values that emphasise individual achievements and independence (Ting-Toomey 2010). People raised in western countries, such as western European and North American countries, usually hold individualist cultures. Individuals are primarily motivated by their own preferences, needs and rights, and the contracts they have established with others. Individuals give priority to their personal goals over the goals of others, and emphasise rational analysis of the advantages and disadvantages of associating with others.

Collectivist cultures endorse collectivist values that rate group achievements higher than individual achievements (Ting-Toomey 2010). People raised in eastern countries, such as Asian, eastern European, some Mediterranean (Greece and Italy), South American and African countries usually hold collectivist cultures. Individuals are actively encouraged to make sacrifices in order to satisfy the group goal. Individuals are primarily motivated by the norms of, and duties imposed by, these collectives.

Conditions underpinning cultural competency in cross-cultural communication

Competent cross-cultural communication has three conditions: motivation, English proficiency, and the knowledge or skills to interpret meaning from non-verbal communication (Lund & O'Regan 2010). 'Motivation' refers to attitudes, values and drives that enable positive cross-cultural communication, and it is viewed as the spiritual dimension of competent intercultural communication (Lund & O'Regan 2010). Cross-cultural encounters are usually associated with ambiguity, anxiety and anticipated negative consequences (Ting-Toomey 2010). Therefore, people may try to avoid communicating with those from other cultures, alienate them, or prevent them from being included.

English proficiency is the number one factor for effective cross-cultural communication (Xu 2007). In an Australian context, patients from non-English-speaking backgrounds may have a low level of English proficiency. Language barriers affect the patient's capacity to express their symptoms and needs, and to comprehend what health professionals say to them. Nurses should be capable of using effective communication strategies in a cross-cultural situation, and verify information from patients and family carers to avoid errors and mistakes.

Non-verbal communication styles such as the use of silence, and indirect verbal styles and non-verbal behaviours such as touch, facial expression, eye movement and body posture are also strongly influenced by culture (Giger & Davidhizar 2008).

People raised in collectivist cultures tend to use silence to indicate disagreement, rather than directly saying 'no'. Saying 'no' directly to a person, particularly to the senior or authority figure is viewed as rude behaviour and is associated with interpersonal conflict. They usually use 'we' instead of 'I' in communication. They do not usually call the person by their first name, but use the title and surname to show their respect, especially when the person is the senior or authority figure. They may use nodding and smiling as signs of respect or greeting, rather than agreements and acceptance. When the nurse pronounces the patient's name and the patient responds with a nod during medication administration, the nurse needs to be aware that the patient may be greeting the nurse, rather than agreeing with the nurse in regard to his or her name.

Learning communication patterns used by different cultural groups is necessary for safe practice. However, you need to be aware of acculturation and its impact on the communication pattern for individuals. Again, making assumptions about a patient's communication style without validating it through nursing assessment is associated with a stereotypical approach to cross-cultural communication that threatens the effective communication and patient–nurse therapeutic relationships.

Cross-cultural communication in multicultural teams

Communication was identified by immigrant nurses from non-English-speaking backgrounds (NESB) as the most challenging aspect of their work (Xu 2007; Xiao et al. 2013). It takes a long time for immigrant nurses to adapt their own communication style to that of the host country or to understand all the nuances of the English language. Studies reveal the use of language is limited by culture, suggesting language proficiency cannot be achieved by study alone, but by interacting with native speakers in a supportive environment (Ting-Toomey 2010). Most immigrant nurses from NESB learn English in their home countries and rely on English dictionaries to interpret meanings of words. They may not be able to comprehend connotative and denotative meanings of words used by patients and colleagues in a sociocultural context (Xu 2007). Therefore, in cross-cultural communication, Australian-born nurses should avoid using slang. Nurses from NESB should be self-aware that errors and mistakes can be easily generated from cross-cultural communication and use every strategy to enhance communication. Australian-born nurses who work side by side with immigrant nurses need to act both as culture brokers and language advisers to facilitate cross-cultural communication in the best interests of patient care.

Refer to the box below to review some tips in cross-cultural communication.

Box 4.1   Tips in cross-cultural communication

Tips in patient–nurse intercultural communication

In intercultural situations, the nurse should always confirm and verify the patient's identity, complaints, requests and needs with the patient, or the patient's relatives, carers or other informants if there is any doubt about the information the nurse has received from the patient. Guidelines recommended by Dr Giger in communicating with patients from NESB are listed below (Giger & Davidhizar 2008, p. 31):

- Use a caring tone of voice and facial expressions to help alleviate the patient's fear.
- Speak slowly and distinctly, but not loudly.
- Use gestures, pictures, and play-acting to help the patient understand.
- Repeat the message in different ways, if necessary.
- Be alert to words the patient seems to understand and use them frequently.
- Keep messages simple and repeat them frequently.
- Avoid using medical terms and abbreviations that the patient may not understand.
- Use an appropriate language dictionary.
- Use interpreters to improve communication.
- Ask the interpreter to translate the message, not just the individual words.
- Obtain feedback to confirm understanding.
- Use an interpreter who is culturally sensitive.

Tips in nurse–nurse intercultural communication

Both Australian-born and immigrant nurses should be aware of cultural differences in communication. They should not interpret a nod, a smile or a 'yes' answer as agreement or acceptance, but use reporting back or asking for feedback as strategies to confirm whether the other person understands their message. Miscommunication in a care team can have fatal consequences in patient care. Tips in nurse–nurse cross-cultural communication identified from the author's research projects (Xiao et al. 2013), as listed below, help nurses avoid errors and mistakes:

- Value diversity in the workplace, and demonstrate by learning and tolerating each other's communication styles and nonverbal behaviours.
- Be willing to modify your own communication style or make allowances in order to reach understanding.
- Establish standard procedures and formats in phone communication, handover and written reporting.
- Use a report-back strategy or obtain feedback to confirm that a nurse has comprehended the message from colleagues.
- Use written and text messages to assist verbal communication if a person's accent affects understanding.
- In order to avoid being misunderstood, Australian-born nurses should avoid slang when communicating with immigrant nurses.

Critical reflection

Use the 'National competency standards for registered nurses' to guide group discussions:

- In your study group, reflect on the cross-cultural experiences you may have had with patients during your clinical placements. Now discuss how you will demonstrate culturally and linguistically appropriate care using standard 2.1, Practices in accordance with the nursing profession's code of ethics and conduct, as a guide.
- Some of you may have experienced communication difficulties in cross-cultural encounters in your clinical placements. What kind of communication strategies have you used to improve cross-cultural communication and avoid misunderstandings? Please check if these communication strategies you have used reflect standard 9.2, Communicate effectively with individuals/groups to facilitate provision of care.
- Have you used online transcultural resources to improve culturally and linguistically appropriate care? Search the web to see if you are able to identify Cue Cards Communication Tool, Communication Board (Eastern Health 2013) and Touch Voice i-Pad. These are useful in assisting patient–nurse intercultural communication and maintaining activities of daily living.

Cultural Competence Development through Daily Practice

As a nurse, you are required to demonstrate culturally competent care for patients by integrating knowledge, skills and attitudes in cross-cultural care in daily practice. Culturally competent care for patients should be demonstrated throughout the entire nursing process, including undertaking culturally and linguistically appropriate nursing assessment, developing a care plan, implementing the care plan and evaluating the care outcomes. Informed by principles of transcultural nursing and cultural safety, you need to work with patients and their families or significant others to identify the care needs associated with a patient's culture and language use. You also need to avoid making assumptions about a patient's culture and communication style, but validate these through nursing assessment. You need to empower patients or their families and significant others to participate in the nursing process so you can achieve culturally and linguistically appropriate care, and determine patient safety and quality of care from the patient's perspective.

The following case study simulates daily care practice in a hospital setting and provides you with an opportunity to discuss how to apply knowledge, skills and attitudes of patient care in cross-cultural encounters.

THEORY TO PRACTICE

Case study: Mr George Dermis's hospital journey

Mr George Dermis, an 85-year-old Greek man, was admitted to a busy general medical ward following a fall at home. He spoke very limited English and his daughter, Mrs Vicki Solomos, was bilingual and the nominated contact person. Mr Dermis was diagnosed with dementia five years ago. RN Mary King, who specialises in geriatric nursing, completed a geriatric-specific assessment on admission. She used the Greek version of the Rowland Universal Dementia Assessment Scale (RUDAS) to test Mr Dermis's current cognitive state. Mr Dermis's RUDAS score was 16 out of 30 (a normal score is 23 or above). In an interview, Vicki told Mary that her father sometimes showed behaviours such as placing things in the wrong place or resisting Vicki's help. Mr Dermis also had hypertension and diabetes, and was on medications for these conditions. Mr Dermis was continent but needed assistance to go to the toilet. He was unable to choose his clothing and needed assistance to dress. He was able to feed himself if Vicki assisted by cutting the meal into small pieces. He also needed Vicki's assistance to drink. Mr Dermis had been using respite care, provided by a local Greek community health care service, one day a week for two years.

Mary also interviewed Vicki about Mr Dermis's life history. Mr Dermis came to Australia 60 years ago from Greece and had only achieved an education up to year 3 in a Greek primary school. He was a factory worker for a local car manufacturing company before his retirement, and had lived with his wife Des for 60 years until Des passed away a year ago. Vicki was the only child of her parents. Mr Dermis moved to Vicki's house and had been cared for by Vicki and her husband since his wife's death. Vicki's husband usually took Mr Dermis walking in the morning in a nearby park. Mr Dermis has three adult grandchildren who are all loving and supportive.

On the night of the admission RN Linda Woods, a first-year graduate nurse, found that Mr Dermis had urinated on the floor and tried to get into another patient's bed. Later, Linda found Mr Dermis lying on the floor with the bedside chair on its side. When she approached Mr Dermis, he yelled something very loudly in Greek that she could not understand. Linda did an assessment and believed that Mr Dermis had not sustained an injury. She was able to get him back onto his bed, but with some problems. When Linda and EN Jan Neil tried to help Mr Dermis back to his bed he was resistant and tried to push them away. Linda reported Mr Dermis's behaviours to the doctor, who prescribed Alprazolam 0.5 mg t.i.d to help Mr Dermis settle down.

Mr Dermis's condition deteriorated over the next two days. On day three, when Vicki visited her father in the morning, she found him confused, and he kept asking her where he was, what time it was and who she was. He was incontinent of urine and was wearing an incontinence pad.

Discussion Questions

1. Based on the information given, what health conditions did Mr Dermis have?
2. Why did RN Mary King use the Greek version of the Rowland Universal Dementia Assessment Scale (RUDAS) to test Mr Dermis's current cognitive state?
3. What environmental modifications can nurses make to improve the quality of care for Mr Dermis?
4. What communication strategies can nurses use in order to identify and meet Mr Dermis's needs?

SUMMARY

Cultural competence is a professional obligation to provide quality care, which involves an effective and efficient response to the care needs of all people, whether they belong to a minority or a majority cultural group. Culturally competent care is both a legal and moral requirement of nurses. In culturally competent care, the provider attends to the total context of the patient's situation, in order to meet the complex cultural healthcare needs of a given individual, family or community. Fundamentally holistic, patient-centred care should underpin nursing care practice. When this is integrated with cultural sensitivity, cultural understanding, cultural knowledge and cultural safety in your daily professional practice, you can then be confident that you are working towards culturally competent care and can achieve equality in health outcomes, irrespective of the type of health services required.

Discussion questions

1. What important concepts do you believe you have learned from this chapter?
2. How will you apply the knowledge to your patient–nurse and nurse–nurse cross-cultural encounters?
3. How prepared are you to deliver culturally and linguistically appropriate care in patient–nurse cross-cultural interactions? What else do you need to know?
4. Imagine that you were admitted to a hospital in a foreign country, where the culture and language differ from yours. What are your expectations of culturally and linguistically appropriate care for nurses?
5. Although most healthcare organisations require employees to wear identification badges and name tags, what flexibility do you have in self-expression or expression of your cultural identify?
6. What types of healthcare access disparities exist for people of CALD background in Australia?

TAHEREH ZIAIAN AND LILY DONGXIA XIAO

Further Reading

Department of Health and Ageing 2012, *National ageing and aged care strategy for people from culturally and linguistically diverse (CALD) backgrounds.* Canberra: Department of Health and Ageing, Online available via: http://www.health.gov.au/internet/main/publishing.nsf/Content/ageing-cald-national-aged-care-strategy-html

Guilherme, M, Glaser, E & García, CM (eds.) 2010, *The intercultural dynamics of multicultural working,* Multilingual Matters, Bristol.

Newman-Giger, J, 2013, *Transcultural nursing: assessment and intervention,* Elsevier Mosby, St. Louis.

NHMRC 2006, *Cultural competency in health: a guide for policy, partnerships and participation.* Canberra: Commonwealth of Australia: National Health and Medical Research Council, Online available via: http://www.nhmrc.gov.au/_files_nhmrc/publications/attachments/hp19.pdf

Australian Transcultural Mental Health Network: www.mmha.org.au

Useful websites

Eastern Health. 2013, *Cue Cards Communication Tool* [Online]. Box Hill, Victoria, Australia Eastern Health. Available: http://www.easternhealth.org.au/services/cuecards/default.aspx#cuecards.

Transcultural Nursing Society 2012, *It is time to celebrate, reflect and look into the future* [Online]. Transcultural Nursing Society. Available: http://www.tcns.org/Foundress.html.

Australian Government's National Health and Medical Research Council (NHMRC) 2006, Cultural competency in health: A guide for policy, partnerships and participation. Available: http://www.nhmrc.gov.au/_files_nhmrc/publications/attachments/hp19.pdf.

References

AIHW 2009, *Nursing and midwifery labour force 2007,* Canberra, Australian Institute of Health and Welfare (AIHW).

Alzheimers' Australia 2011, *Timely diagnosis of dementia: can we do better? A report for Alzheimer's Australia paper 24,* Alzheimer's Australia, Canberra.

Australian Bureau of Statistics 2012, *Cultural diversity in Australia,* Australian Bureau of Statistics, Canberra.

Campesino, M 2008, 'Beyond transculturalism: critiques of cultural education in nursing', *Journal of Nursing Education* vol. 47(7) pp. 298–304.

Commonwealth of Australia 1999, *Australian multiculturalism for a new century: towards inclusiveness: a report by the National Multicultural Advisory Council.*

Cross, T, Bazron, B et al. 1989, *Towards a culturally competent system of care,* Washington, DC, National Technical Assistance Center for Children's Mental Health, Georgetown University Child Development Center, vol. I.

Department of Health and Ageing 2012, *National ageing and aged care strategy for people from culturally and linguistically diverse (CALD) backgrounds*, Department of Health and Ageing, Canberra.

Department of Immigration and Citizenship 2011, *The people of Australia: Australia's multicultural policy*.

Department of Immigration and Citizenship 2013, *Access and equity*, Canberra.

Department of Immigration and Citizenship 2013, *Fact sheet 15: Population growth*, Canberra.

Dreachslin, JL, Hunt, PL et al. 2000 'Workforce diversity: implications for the effectiveness of health care delivery teams', *Social Science & Medicine* vol. 50(10), pp. 1403–14.

Eastern Health 2013, *Cue cards communication tool*. Retrieved 20 January 2013, http://www.easternhealth.org.au/services/cuecards/default.aspx#cuecards.

Giger, JN 2013, *Transcultural nursing: assessment and intervention*, Elsevier Mosby, St Louis.

Giger, JN & Davidhizar, R 2008, *Transcultural nursing: assessment and intervention*, 5th edn., Mosby, St Louis.

Jeong, SYS, Hickey, N et al 2011, 'Understanding and enhancing the learning experiences of culturally and linguistically diverse nursing students in an Australian bachelor of nursing program', *Nurse Education Today* vol. 31(3), pp. 238–44.

Johnstone, M & Kanitsaki, O 2005, *Cultural safety and cultural competence in health care and nursing: an Australian study*, RMIT University, Melbourne.

Leininger, MM 2006, 'Culture care diversity and universality theory and evolution of the ethnonursing method' in MM Leininger & MR McFarland (eds) *Culture care diversity and universality: a worldwide nursing theory*, 2nd edn, MA, Jones and Bartlett, Sudbury, pp. 1–42.

Lund, DA and O'Regan, JP 2010, 'National occupational standards in intercultural working: models of theory and assessment', in M Guilherme, E Glaser & MdC Mendez-Garcia (eds), *The intercultural dynamics of multicultural working*, Bristol, UK, Multilingual Matters, pp. 41–58.

NHMRC 2006, *Cultural competency in health: a guide for policy, partnerships and participation*. Canberra, Commonwealth of Australia: National Health and Medical Research Council.

Nursing and Midwifery Board of Australia 2010, *National competency standards for the registered nurse*.

Nursing Council of New Zealand 2011, *Guidelines for cultural safety, the Treaty of Waitangi and Maori health in nursing education and practice*.

Office of Minority Health 2013, *National culturally and linguistically appropriate services standards in health and health care final report*, US Department of Health and Human Services Office of Minority Health, Washington, DC.

Papadopoulos, I 2006, *Transcultural health and social care: development of culturally competent practitioners*, Elsevier, London.

Purnell, L 2011, 'Models and theories focused on culture', in JB Butts, & KL Rich (eds.) *Philosophies and theories for advanced nursing practice*, Jones and Bartlett, Sudbury MA, chapter 22, pp. 525–68.

Salamonson, Y, Ramjan, L et al. 2012, 'Diversity and demographic heterogeneity of Australian nursing students: a closer look', *International Nursing Review* vol. 59(1), pp. 59–65.

Ting-Toomey, S 1999, *Communicating across cultures*, Guilford Press, New York.

Ting-Toomey, S 2010, 'Intercultural conflict interaction competence: from theory to practice' in M Guilherme, E Glaser & MdC Mendez-Garcia (eds), *The intercultural dynamics of multicultural working*, Multilingual Matters, Bristol, UK, pp. 21–40.

Transcultural Nursing Society 2012, *It is time to celebrate, reflect and look into the future* Retrieved 10/12/2013, from http://www.tcns.org/Foundress.html.

Xiao, L D, Willis, E et al. 2014, 'Factors affecting the integration of immigrant nurses into the nursing workforce: a double hermeneutic study', *International Journal of Nursing Studies* vol. 51(4), pp. 640–653.

Xu, Y 2007, 'Strangers in strange lands: a metasynthesis of lived experiences of immigrant Asian nurses working in western countries', *Advances in Nursing Science* vol. 30(3), pp. 246–65.

Entering Clinical Settings

5

BARBARA PARKER, ANGELA KUCIA AND LUCY HOPE

LEARNING OBJECTIVES

After reading this chapter, you will be able to:

- discuss the employer's expectations of the registered nurse role
- begin planning your career in nursing
- develop a professional relationship with your preceptor
- apply the principles of experiential learning to your nursing practice
- identify your ongoing learning needs as you move into the registered nurse role.

KEY TERMS

Clinical assessment
Clinical placement
Curriculum vitae
Experiential learning
Infection control
Preceptorship
Risk
Time management
Transition to Professional Practice Program (TPPP)

Transition from University to the Clinical Setting

The transition from university to the clinical setting is an opportunity to put into practice new knowledge and skills. Clinical placements prepare students for the final transition to the workplace and the registered nurse role. There are many support systems available to help you navigate this transition. In this chapter, we look at these supports and examine what you need to consider before clinical placements and when you undertake the **Transition to Professional Practice Program (TPPP)** as a new graduate.

TRANSITION TO PROFESSIONAL PRACTICE PROGRAM (TPPP) — A 12-month employment opportunity with scheduled professional learning activities and experiences that supports and enables the graduate nurse to adapt to the RN role.

Prior Work Experience

As a nursing student, you have already gained experience from many different sources, and will be expected to bring all of this to your subsequent employment as a registered nurse. During secondary school, you may have undertaken part-time paid work, for instance in a retail or customer service environment. If you entered your nursing course straight after school, you may have continued with this part-time work during your undergraduate nursing degree program. Many young people gain experience in management roles in part-time jobs, for instance working as shift supervisors or assistant managers. Thus, part-time employment provides opportunities for you to gain valuable skills, such as time-management and communication, that are transferable to the healthcare sector. Many nursing students do not recognise that these skills can be used to help succeed in a nursing career. Alternatively, now might be the time to consider a part-time role in healthcare to assist you in transferring your new knowledge to practice.

If you are a mature-aged student, you may be coming to nursing as your second or even third career and, again, your experience is invaluable to your potential new role. Often, you have substantial financial commitments and established full-time or part-time careers in other employment fields. Combining this with study is challenging, as nursing demands a large commitment to study, on-campus activities and clinical placements. While existing career roles do provide you with essential skills that can be transferred to the healthcare setting, you can also benefit from shifting to a healthcare role during study.

Working in healthcare while studying

Universities recognise that students need to work to support themselves during their courses. When you are considering your employment choices, take every opportunity to immerse yourself in the nursing profession. Remember that at the end of your degree you will be working as a registered nurse and it makes sense to make the move into the field as soon as possible. Working in health will help you:

TIME MANAGEMENT – Organising and prioritising workloads within the time available.

- gain **time management** skills
- hone fundamental nursing skills such as assessment, skin care and hygiene
- learn how the healthcare system works, from inpatient to community services
- increase confidence in your own practice (Alsup et al. 2006).

Working in a healthcare environment offers you plenty of opportunity for practice, and, if you pick the right workplace, you will be supported in taking time off for study, examinations and clinical placements. It is advisable to discuss this at the interview.

Major public and private hospitals offer employment positions for nursing students in the second and third years of their program. Depending on the curriculum you are studying, you may be offered an assistant in nursing (AIN) position during second year, but the majority of venues offer this position to third-year students. This is because third-year students usually have a more established knowledge and skill base and can practise at an advanced student level. At second-year level, you may be able to secure a personal care attendant (PCA) role in an acute care setting, without undertaking additional qualifications such as a Certificate III. In addition, from the first year of a program, many students are employed as PCAs in aged care facilities. These positions may also require some additional training, either by the institution or in the form of a vocational education and training (VET) qualification.

PCA and AIN positions are advertised in the careers sections of newspapers and on careers websites, or you can approach the nursing administration department of the organisation in which you would like to work. Treat this like any other interview process and, before you apply for a position, make sure you prepare adequately by following these steps:

1. Research the organisation. Get a sense of the vision and mission of the organisation, the type of clients it caters for, and the care that is provided.
2. Find out the name of the director of care/nursing or the recruitment officer.
3. Write or update your **curriculum vitae**. If you need help with this, your university careers department should be able to assist.
4. Compile essential documentation such as criminal history clearance, senior first aid certificate, including current CPR, and immunisation information.
5. Gather evidence and records of your clinical practice, for instance evidence that you have completed manual handling, **infection control** or blood safe modules, and so on.

Experiential learning refers to the process of learning through practical experience, such as that you receive in your clinical placements. It prepares you for your future role in complex and changing work environments. It enables deep and applied learning within the context of practice (Kolb et al. 2000). Formal placements within healthcare settings are essential to learning safe practice, and should provide outcomes that give you clear guidelines for staged improvement across a program and constructive feedback that will assist in learning. Clinical placements enhance lifelong learning, capability and professionalism, and provide opportunities to transfer, reorganise, apply, synthesise and evaluate knowledge (Cope et al. 2000; Levett-Jones et al. 2006).

Within undergraduate nursing programs there are many formal placement opportunities to gain experience and interact with clients in the community,

CURRICULUM VITAE (CV)— A summary of one's attributes for employment, including educational and employment history and qualifications.

INFECTION CONTROL — Actions taken to prevent nosocomial or healthcare-associated infection.

EXPERIENTIAL LEARNING — Making meaning from direct experience to build knowledge; e.g. the knowledge acquired during clinical placement.

aged care facilities, the acute care sector and other specialty environments. Some nursing programs expose students to the clinical setting in the first semester of the program, while others delay this until students have a broad knowledge base from which to practise. This latter approach is strengthened by informal experiential learning activities that expose students to healthy people across the lifespan so that fundamental nursing skills, such as assessment, can be mastered. In addition, simulation, role play and interactive online activities are used in the learning environment. This is a non-threatening way for you to practise new skills in an environment where getting it wrong is an opportunity for learning, not a punitive experience.

Students are rigorously assessed in the clinical environment. Assessment occurs under the supervision of clinical preceptors and a clinical facilitator usually employed by the university. At times, it may feel that you are under a microscope and every staff member is keeping an eye on your practice, but clinical placements can be a very positive experience. Nursing staff welcome students into their work areas, and many nurses are very keen to provide you with additional support. Official support roles include those of the clinical facilitator (or clinical lecturer) and the preceptor.

The role of the clinical facilitator is to ensure that you meet the course objectives and maintain the standards of nursing practice. They are there to mentor, support and assess students on placement. They may not take on a teaching role, and you can expect to see them about two to three times per week. The clinical facilitator may be seconded from the venue—that is, they normally work at the venue as a nurse but are given time off to undertake the facilitation role—or they may be an external person employed by the university. Either way, the clinical facilitator's role is to advocate for you and ensure that an environment exists in which you can achieve your learning objectives. In many programs the facilitator also undertakes all of the **clinical assessments** and is an excellent resource if you are having difficulty with any of these.

The preceptor is a registered nurse with whom you are paired, who provides additional mentoring, guidance and support at each point of the day. Nursing students will often be rostered on with the preceptor so that they can work alongside each other. In this way, the preceptor provides a teaching and support role while still attending to their usual patient workload.

CLINICAL ASSESSMENT – An evaluation of a person's state of health based upon the person's medical history, physical examination, and results of associated laboratory tests.

Critical reflection

You are assigned to a busy surgical unit for your first acute care specialty placement. During week 2 of the placement you are allocated to work with a number of different registered nurse (RN) preceptors and you feel you have had little time to build a rapport with any staff member. While undertaking a medication round, the registered nurse is called away and he asks you to give the oral medication you have just been checking to the patient in bed 4, which you do. On his return, the registered nurse resumes the round and you check another medication. This time, the patient's folder is requested by the doctor and, being short of time, the registered nurse elects to administer the medication to the patient without the patient's folder. You are the second person checking this medication.

- What do you say to the registered nurse?
- Is the correct procedure being followed here?
- What is the student nurse's scope of practice with regard to medication administration?
- What support systems are in place for students in this situation?

Preparing for placement

In order to be ready to engage fully in the **clinical placement**, you need to have a broad knowledge base and have had the opportunity to undertake some skill practice, role-play and simulation activities at university. It is important that you engage as much as possible with these opportunities and with the university environment. People will talk about the clinical setting as the 'real world', but students inhabit many 'real' worlds. These include home, work and recreation, which all impact on the amount of time a student spends on their university study. Students sometimes parrot the saying that 'Ps get degrees'. A 'P' is the minimum required to pass a course and as such is an acceptable grade. However, what a 'P' really means is that instead of knowing half of what you need to know, you actually *don't know* half of what is vitally important for your safe practice. This, in turn, has a profound effect on your patients' outcomes. It also affects your overall grade point average (GPA) and, in a competitive postgraduate employment environment, achieving as high a GPA as possible will impress future employers. Your theory courses are essential learning for your clinical placements, and you should apply yourself wholeheartedly to your study. An understanding of pathophysiology, pharmacology, sociology, primary healthcare, law and ethics, quality and safety is essential to you being able to adequately assess and manage your clients' care.

CLINICAL PLACEMENT — A period of time spent in a health setting where the student has an opportunity to integrate knowledge and practical skills with the goal of meeting specific clinical objectives relevant to a particular course.

Essential criteria

Make sure you are aware of your university's policy regarding uniforms, name badges and essential documentation. All healthcare settings in Australia require students to produce a criminal history clearance, so your university will require this before they can place you in a venue. Some states require additional documentation, such as a blue card, 'Working with children' check or placement orientation checklist from the health department in your state.

In addition, your immunisation status is important, and you should consult your general practitioner or local government immunisation service to be screened and immunised for infectious diseases, as recommended in *The Australian immunisation handbook*, tenth edition (Department of Health and Ageing & National Health and Medical Research Council 2013). You should also check that all other standard childhood immunisations are up to date for the state in which you are attending the healthcare venue. To assist you in this, government websites in each state provide information about immunisation guidelines for healthcare workers.

In order to be able to place you in the clinical setting, many universities also require a current senior first-aid certificate with annual cardio-pulmonary resuscitation (CPR) updates. Your university will have this information online. Some items may take some time to complete, so make sure you are aware of your requirements early in the program.

Orientation

Either before placement begins or on the first day, you can expect an orientation to the venue and the ward in which you will be working. Among other things, it is essential that you understand where the emergency exits are located and what sounds signify danger or an emergency, and that you are familiar with the infection control and manual handling procedures of the venue. The orientation will also outline your responsibilities as a student, including what shifts you will work, what time shifts start and finish, who your preceptor is, how long your breaks are and when you can take them, the rules relating to when you can leave the ward, and who to call if you are going to be off sick. Some venues may require you to undertake a CPR and manual handling update, which is an excellent opportunity for further learning and practice in these essential skills.

Learning objectives

Be sure you understand how you will be assessed and compile relevant documentation before you start your placement. If you are unsure of where to find any of this information, seek advice from your lecturer or course coordinator. Students are expected to arrive at placement with some idea of what they wish to achieve during this time. Think about the skills you have studied and practised at university and are really keen to put into practice. Think not only of tasks such as 'setting up an intravenous therapy line' or 'showering a patient' but also about your time management and communication skills. In preparing these objectives, consider also how you will prove that you are performing these skills well. Your ability to devise strategies and collect evidence of your safe practices will help your clinical facilitator provide ongoing feedback and evaluation, assess your competency to practise and decide on your grade.

Reflecting on practice

Working with different nurses can help you determine what sort of nurse you want to be (Bradbury-Jones, et al. 2009). Critically appraise others and their work, and determine if the behaviour(s) and practice(s) you observe are what you would incorporate into your safe practice. Or are they examples of what *not* to do?

Measuring performance

Most clinical assessments are competency-based. These competencies have been accepted as the standards by which we measure safe practice. The benefits of using competencies in clinical assessment are that you can clearly identify what you should be doing and how to achieve it. You will need to know and understand the NMBA's *National competency standards for the registered nurse* (NMBA 2006, Appendix E) and/or *National competency standards for the midwife* (NMBA & Australian College of Midwives 2006). These are available on the Nursing and Midwifery regulatory board website.

Competency-based assessment on clinical placement:

- emphasises the importance of clinical practice, in addition to theory, in learning outcomes
- stimulates student learning
- recognises student excellence
- provides measurable outcomes
- provides evidence to support the university policies regarding assessment
- provides future employers with evidence of skills (a more effective way of communicating with employers)
- facilitates the move away from task-oriented clinical practice.

Apart from your clinical skills, professional practice requires a number of other skills. You will also be assessed on your organisation, time management, critical thinking and problem-solving abilities. Some strategies for meeting your learning needs on clinical placement include:

- If you don't know something—*ask*. You are not expected to know everything. You are expected to have a beginner's knowledge base and to use this to ask appropriate questions.

- Consider what resources are available for you to begin finding solutions to things you don't know. These resources may include:
  - registered nurses, enrolled nurses and care workers
  - medical officers
  - policy and procedure manuals—digital and hard copy
  - journals, texts
  - other students
  - your clinical facilitator
  - websites (remember to use only official and reliable websites for healthcare information).
- Provide suggested solutions to problems you identify.
- Understand the link between theory (including anatomy and physiology) and practice, and be able to articulate this.
- Provide a rationale for nursing care—why are you doing this?
- If you have not had the opportunity to undertake an activity or skill in the clinical setting, then this is okay. Explain to your preceptor that you understand the theory that underpins the practice and have practised in the simulation environment. Ask if you can observe the preceptor undertake the task and then supervise you doing it. Request that you are notified the next time there is an opportunity to do the task.
- Provide a list of skills and activities to your preceptor that will help you meet your learning objectives. If possible, put this list in the nurses' station and ask the rest of the staff to let you know if any opportunities for these arise.

Critical reflection

You are in the third year of your undergraduate nursing program. You have just begun your last clinical placement. So far in your program, you have had placements in aged care and paediatrics, and a rural placement in a mixed medical/surgical ward. Your current placement is in a busy emergency department (ED) in a hospital that you have not worked in before. You have just finished your orientation to the department and this is your second shift in the ED. You are working a late shift on a Saturday night and the department is over capacity, with long waiting times to be seen. You are doing your best to assist everyone, but you are feeling out of your depth and unsupported, as everyone is so busy. When the team leader (TL) comes to you for the third time and tells you to do something that is beyond your experience, you explain that you have not done this before and will need supervision. The TL rolls her eyes and says that she hasn't got time to do it for you, and asks you what you learned at university that is of any use.

- How would you respond in this situation?
- Are there any strategies you can think of that you could put in place to avoid this type of situation in the future?

Personal considerations

Most students have a wonderful, exciting clinical experience. It is normal to feel anxious in the early days at a new clinical placement, but with support from facilitators and preceptors this soon settles. The first week of the first placement is a particularly vulnerable time, and students should try to reduce other life stressors at this time. Students want to do well and, above all, they want to do no harm, and this can contribute to putting enormous pressure on themselves. This stress can manifest in different ways: some students may find that they become tearful or irritable, sometimes forgetful or vulnerable to illness (Elliott 2002; Yonge et al. 2002). There is no doubt that the clinical experience is tiring for students, because of both shift work and stress, and you need to ensure that you are getting adequate rest and sleep, good nutrition and exercise to sustain energy levels. For some students, the added stress at this time means that they need additional support beyond what can be provided by the venue or academic staff. Universities offer counselling services and learning advisers who can help with strategies for coping and for assessments, so familiarise yourself with these services.

Before you applied for your degree, you should have planned to ensure that you could meet the requirements of the program. You should know how much time you need to commit to study, how long and when your clinical placements are, and when and for how long you are expected on campus. This will help you to plan your work and family commitments to ensure that you are available for all aspects of your program. When you are planning, be sure to factor in time for rest, for family and for fun. Be realistic about what you can achieve and talk to your institution about a part-time study plan if needed. It may take a little longer but you will maximise your opportunity to gain the knowledge and experience you require to complete the degree and emerge as a safe novice practitioner.

When you have finished your placement, make sure that you keep all originals of your placement assessment items. Employers will request these when you apply for your TPPP. Remember that all the information you collected during your placements, such as strategies and evidence to show that you meet the competencies, can be used in your application and interview to prove that you are capable of meeting the standards of safe practice. This, together with a high grade point average (GPA) will be important in securing the venue of your choice.

BARBARA PARKER, ANGELA KUCIA AND LUCY HOPE

THEORY TO PRACTICE

Communication and teamwork

Throughout my nursing program we attended clinical skill sessions within a custom-designed on campus simulation unit. Each session we listened to handover and received our allocation to a simulated patient. We greeted the 'patient' with 'Good morning Mr ... my name is ... and I will be looking after you today'. In our minds the patient always responded politely and we set about assessing, planning and prioritising care. During each activity the 'patient' was mute except for the occasional cough, wheeze or moan. At the end of each session we said our goodbyes and left feeling pleased with ourselves and the excellent care we had provided. My first formal clinical placement allocation was to a residential aged care facility. On my first day I was paired with a personal care attendant (PCA) who barely acknowledged my existence. I trailed along behind her feeling upset and isolated. We entered the room of a very frail older woman and I waited for the PCA to give her a greeting and introduce me. Instead the PCA immediately began preparing the hygiene equipment and I approached the resident. I started with the usual 'Good morning Mrs....' and expected a pleasant response. To my surprise and discomfort the resident became quite distressed and began shouting at me to get away. The PCA also shouted at me to leave the resident alone and move out of the way. I tried to assist the situation by calming the resident but I was not able to and in the end I had to concede that the PCA probably understood the situation better than me. I had learned about communication and therapeutic relationships with clients at university and practised weekly on my 'patients' in 'the simulated environment. I thought this prepared me to interact well with clients in the clinical setting, but communicating with a real person is a lot different. I didn't have the experience to help me to anticipate problems or variations that may arise in communicating with an unwell or cognitively impaired client in the clinical setting, and the need to plan around these factors. I now understood why I needed to undertake a good assessment, consider my client's history and presenting characteristics, and speak to other staff and/or family who knew the person better than I to reduce the risk of an unfavourable reaction. I also understood how important teamwork is and that treating colleagues with kindness and respect also assists in a better outcome for clients.

Discussion Questions

Consider the situation above.

1. What actions/strategies can the student include next time to prevent this type of situation?
2. What is the role of the student in improving communication and teamwork?
3. What internal and external support systems are available to the student in this situation?
4. Are there occupational health and safety issues involved in this example?

Career Goals

Even before you began your program, you may have had some idea of where you wanted to finish up. If you don't, don't worry, as you have plenty of time to make these decisions. Many students are still not sure at graduation, and the transition year is a good time to look at what specialty areas are available.

One of your early goals should be to work hard to gain a high GPA and good clinical assessments. Although nurses are still in demand, employers will want to take the best graduates, and these markers of your ability to practise safely will assist you to gain the TPPP of your choice.

The third year of your program is a good time to start seriously thinking about your career goals and aspirations, and positioning yourself to meet them. Use the clinical placements as a time to seek out the knowledge and expertise of registered nurses and find out what areas are available for you to work in once you complete your degree. At university, talk with your lecturers, program directors and counselling staff, as these people have experience in the clinical area and in assisting students gain employment. Your university should also have a career centre that can assist in compiling curriculum vitae, applying for positions, interview skills and more.

Your longer term goals should be built around lifelong learning, and a high GPA will position you to take up further study opportunities. Some of these opportunities include specialising in your area of practice through Graduate Certificates, Graduate Diplomas, Masters or Nurse Practitioner programs. In addition, evidence-based practice requires excellent research skills, and you may consider an Honours research program, leading to a PhD.

Transition to Professional Practice Program

The transition from student to registered nurse is a major milestone. You have been working towards this goal for some time but, initially, being a graduate nurse may seem a bit daunting. Most newly graduated nurses will undertake TPPP. According to Levett-Jones and Fitzgerald (2005), transition programs share three primary goals:
1. to develop competent and confident registered nurses
2. to facilitate professional adjustment
3. to develop commitment to a career in nursing.

For the majority of nurses, the TPPP is a hospital-based program that takes place over a twelve-month period. During this time, the graduate nurse has an opportunity to work in different ward environments, with the aim of applying the knowledge, theories and experiences obtained during university studies to the nursing management of particular patient populations and clinical situations. During the TPPP year, the graduate nurse also learns to deal with relationship issues with patients and their families, as well as with other members of the healthcare team, including nursing colleagues. As a graduate nurse, you will have many new experiences. You will have an opportunity to apply and further develop the critical thinking skills that underpinned your nursing undergraduate studies.

Adapting to a new role and a new working environment

The TPPP year is challenging and sometimes stressful, but it is exciting too. This may be your first experience of paid employment, and the transition from student to paid employee is likely very welcome from a financial perspective. Shift work and working at weekends may take some getting used to, and you will need to structure your social life around your work commitments. Fortunately, most employers are aware of the importance of retaining nurse employees and many offer flexible shift patterns.

Healthcare is constantly evolving and changing due to technological advances, increasing economic pressures and public expectations. A nursing career involves lifelong learning to keep up to date with new evidence and changes in practice. Although you are no longer a student nurse, you are entering a new stage of your education, and you must be prepared to continue to be involved in active learning.

Working in a hospital, you will become aware that there is a hierarchical administrative structure and complex social system that you will need to learn to work within. You will develop many new relationships at a number of different levels and you will need to adapt to the social aspects of your new environment. You will also need to understand what is expected of you and what resources are available to help you to perform effectively in your role.

Critical reflection

You are a new graduate nurse on your second ward placement in a medical ward. You have started the early shift and are receiving handover for your allocated patients. During handover, the nightshift nurse states that 'Mr Smith has deteriorated overnight, his breathing is shallow and his respiratory rate is low. No observations were taken, as he is for comfort measures only.' However, upon closer inspection of his case notes, you cannot see a clear order indicating Mr Smith's resuscitation status. You promptly attend Mr Smith's bedside and take a set of vital signs and use your assessment skills, which indicate that his consciousness is impaired and he is not responding to verbal or painful stimuli.

- What action(s) would you take?
- Do you need to notify senior staff members? Why?
- Who do you need to clarify the resuscitation status with?
- How can this situation be avoided in future?

Orientation programs

A comprehensive orientation program is important in preparing graduate nurses for their new role, and it is also a key factor in retaining staff (Mayer & Mayer 2000). It is therefore in the best interests of your employer to provide appropriate orientation, and in your interests to seek employment in an organisation that has a good orientation program. Orientation to the organisation usually takes place over a few days, and includes information such as the physical layout of the institution, the departmental and hierarchical structure, core business and organisational values, goals and policies. The importance of organisational values, goals and policies was discussed in Chapter 1. The orientation program may also provide an opportunity to undertake compulsory training sessions such as manual handling, fire safety, basic life support and drug calculation tests.

Preceptorship

It is likely that when you start work in a new ward or clinical setting, a preceptor will be assigned to you. The person undertaking this **preceptorship** role is usually a senior nurse who has had sufficient experience in the clinical setting to be able to act as a role model and resource person for more junior nurses. When starting somewhere new, it is often reassuring to know that there is a person who has agreed to be available to you and assist you in your practice, education and socialisation to your new working environment. Some senior nurses have had educational preparation or in-service education to support their preceptor role, while others may be selected because of their clinical skills and expertise, or expressed willingness to teach junior staff. Usually, the relationship with the preceptor lasts for a few weeks, and it may be that you do not often work on the same shift as your preceptor. The assignment of a preceptor to a new graduate is often somewhat arbitrary, and you may find that you identify another registered nurse on the ward who you find is an appropriate role model for you and who is willing to help and guide you.

PRECEPTORSHIP — The practice of a student/graduate nurse working with an RN in the practice setting to increase the knowledge and skills application of the student/graduate nurse.

Employers' expectations

As you begin your career as a registered nurse, you will find that expectations of you in your role are quite different from those that you encountered as a student.

You need to be aware of what your employer expects of you. Some of these expectations are explicitly stated in the contract that you signed prior to commencing employment, but there may be other expectations that are implicit in the role. It is assumed that the graduate nurse is functioning at the advanced beginner level, with basic levels of competence that require support and guidance for safe practice. New graduates should be aware of their limitations and seek guidance as needed. As adult learners, new graduates are expected to identify their learning needs, and in collaboration with the preceptor, manager and clinical educator, participate in planning learning experiences and goals (Santuci 2004). Graduate nurses are expected to be accountable for their own practice and for developing their own best practice (Santuci 2004). As you have recently been a student, you may be aware of recent developments or changes in practice that may allow you to raise questions or make suggestions in your working environment when you see that practices could be improved or updated in line with current evidence. New perspectives from newcomers can offer fresh ideas for positive change (Santuci 2004). Don't be discouraged if your suggestions for change are not immediately embraced by your colleagues—resistance to change is firmly entrenched in some workplaces. It may take some time and representation of the evidence for change and the benefits to be expected to persuade people to embrace new ideas.

As a healthcare employee, there are a number of expectations regarding professional behaviour and safe practice that apply to almost all work settings, some of which may have ethical and legal aspects.

Access to electronic records and resources

During orientation, you should be provided with an overview of the computer-based systems in use within the organisation. To facilitate this, you should have good general computer skills. You may be expected to use a number of computer programs that are integral to activities such as:

- generating nursing care plans
- recording patient admissions, discharges, transfers and movement within the hospital
- ordering tests and services
- obtaining laboratory and investigative results
- email communication
- accessing library resources.

You will be given passwords in order to access these systems. Before accessing these systems, you will have to acknowledge that you are aware of privacy policies and that you will not access or disclose information inappropriately. Be aware that any activity you undertake in accessing workplace systems is monitored and can be tracked back to you. Therefore, you should ensure that you log out of the system when you complete the necessary activity. You also need to be aware that you are accountable for information that you have input.

Information on the regulation of health privacy in Australia is available from the Australian Government's National Health and Medical Research Council (NHMRC) online at www.nhmrc.gov.au/guidelines/publications/nh53.

Workplace health and safety

An introduction to organisational expectations with regard to workplace health and safety (WHS) is usually part of the orientation program. As an employee, you must agree to comply with the organisation's WHS directives. This is for your own personal safety, and that of other employees and clientele of the organisation.

Most nursing orientation programs have a training session on manual handling. Historically, nurses commonly experienced back injuries as a result of lifting patients. Hospitals now have 'no lifting' policies to prevent these injuries. It is important that you are familiar with organisational manual handling policies and comply with them at all times. Ensure that you know how to safely use manual handling aids and equipment, and that you prepare to undertake annual manual handling updates.

You should not use equipment unless you have been shown how to do so safely. You should also be aware of issues pertaining to electrical safety, particularly in critical care areas, where patients are attached to monitors and often have several infusion pumps and various other medical devices in use. If you find a fault with any equipment, electrical or otherwise, it must be removed from use, the ward manager must be notified, and the equipment should be tagged to alert other ward staff that it is faulty.

Needlestick injuries are another common source of injury for nurses. They are preventable providing that appropriate processes are followed. Blood-borne diseases that could be transmitted by needlestick injuries include human immunodeficiency virus (HIV), hepatitis B (HBV) and hepatitis C (HCV). Information on organisational strategies to reduce the **risk** of needlestick injury should be provided during your orientation program. You should explore policies and procedures for reducing the risk of needlestick injury to yourself and others. Ensure that you know how to dispose safely of sharps, and where sharps containers are located.

RISK – The chance or possibility of an event occurring that will have a negative outcome.

Infection control

Healthcare-associated infections continue to be a major problem for patient safety, and contribute to unexpected patient deaths. They also place a significant burden on healthcare resources (Pittet 2005). The evolution of multi resistant organisms makes some forms of infection difficult to manage. Preventing the spread of infection in the healthcare setting, where patients are often immuno-compromised, is essential. Nurses have an active role in reducing the spread of hospital-acquired infections. In fact, Florence Nightingale was the first person to suggest that nurses could survey hospital-acquired infections (Pittet 2005). Many hospitals have specific policy and procedure manuals for infection control, and may have an infection-control nurse or infection-control team. You should be familiar with infection-control policies and procedures and do everything that you can to prevent the spread of infection. Many healthcare organisations offer vaccination to their staff, to prevent diseases such as hepatitis, tuberculosis, tetanus and influenza. Vaccination against these diseases is in your best interests and the interests of the patients for whom you are caring. You may have been immunised during your undergraduate training, but if not you should consider this as a priority.

A good resource for you to access more information on infection control is the Australian Government's Department of Health and Ageing infection control guidelines, available online at www.health.gov.au/internet/main/publishing.nsf/content/icg-guidelines-index.htm.

Responding to hospital emergencies

Various emergency situations can occur in the hospital setting, and staff must know how to manage them. During your orientation, it is likely that you will undergo some training in how to manage situations such as fire, security threats and medical emergencies. It is important that you know what is expected of you, as a graduate nurse, in these situations. Generally, annual updates are required, and it is your responsibility to ensure that you complete these updates when they are due. You may have had some experience of these updates during your clinical placements.

Shift work

Service industries, such as healthcare, operate over a 24-hour period, and therefore must employ shift workers. Generally, the number of staff on duty outside business hours is kept to a minimum, but it is likely that you will be expected to do rotations of night duty during your graduate year. Shift work disrupts the synchronous relationship between the body's internal clock and the environment, which can affect your general health and feeling of well-being. Physiologic effects include changes in rhythms of core temperature, various hormonal levels, immune functioning, and activity–rest cycles. Problems such as sleep disturbances, increased accidents and injuries and social isolation may result (Berger & Hobbs 2005). It is important that you do what you can to reduce the negative effects of shift work. Schedule six to eight hours of sleep and use power napping before work when needed. Avoid food and drinks that are likely to cause wakefulness, such as alcohol and caffeine, for at least six hours prior to scheduled sleep times.

Developing a sense of belonging

During your TPPP, it is likely that you will have three to four different ward placements. You may have had some input into your ward placements, but the overall goal is to provide you with a range of nursing experiences. Each of your placements may be quite different, and it may take some time to settle in to each. You will enjoy some more than others, and this may be influenced by how supportive your co-workers are. It may help you to decide where you want to work when you complete your TPPP. If you find a ward or workplace that you really enjoy and would like to come back to when you complete your TPPP, let the nurse manager know, as they may then be in a position to advocate for you if a position becomes available.

For some years now there has been a shortage of nurses in most western countries, which means that hospitals, in particular, are employing a larger number of graduate nurses. Some wards depend upon a large cohort of graduate nurses to maintain staffing requirements. Being a new graduate on a ward that has a high percentage of new graduates can have advantages and disadvantages. On the plus side, the staff are accustomed to working with graduate nurses and will understand the need for education, support and mentorship. However, constantly mentoring new staff can be quite exhausting for the permanent staff on a ward, particularly if they have a heavy workload of their own. The staff may feel that once a graduate nurse has reached some level of independence in a particular ward and the need for close supervision is lessened, the graduate nurse is moved to another area and the cycle begins again. Permanent ward staff may feel frustrated that they haven't got time to adequately support new graduate nurses. If this frustration is outwardly expressed, it may leave you feeling inadequate and inept, and this may result in you feeling hesitant about approaching certain ward staff for help. Don't be tempted to undertake a task for which you have not had sufficient experience or practice without guidance or support. If you are not getting the support that you require, you may need to address the problem with the nurse manager.

THEORY TO PRACTICE

Lifting patients

During my nursing training, we were taught how to lift patients with a lifting machine. It didn't seem to be too difficult. I learnt how to operate the machine (although it was a bit technical). We (the student nurses) broke into groups of three and took turns being the patient. We lifted each other using the machine—it was fun, and as far as I was concerned (and the nurse educators, for that matter) I was competent to lift patients! During my first week on the ward, I had to use the lifter to lift a patient from his bed to the chair. He had undergone major abdominal surgery and had intravenous drips, wound drains, a urinary catheter and a huge abdominal wound. I didn't ask the other staff to help me. When I had asked for help on other matters, some of the staff had seemed irritated because they were busy, while others seemed unapproachable. I thought I should be able to do this by myself. When I tried to get the patient into the lifter, he seemed to have a lot of pain and was afraid of falling. He struggled against me, and I was afraid I would dislodge some of his drips or drains in the process of moving him. The result was that we both ended up in a tangle, and I felt very foolish when I had to go and ask the senior registered nurse for help. I found that the reality of lifting a patient in the clinical setting is a lot different from lifting a nurse in the clinical skills lab. Although I had been taught how to use a mechanical lifter, I had not had experience that helped me to anticipate problems or variations that may arise in lifting an unwell patient in the clinical setting, and the need to plan around these factors. I also learnt that the welfare of the patient was far more important than my fear of an unfavourable reaction if I asked for help.

Discussion Questions

Consider the situation above.

1. After reading this chapter and considering the issues with transition from student to graduate nurse, why do you think the nurse may have acted in this way?
2. How do you think this situation might, have been prevented?
3. Are there occupational health and safety issues involved in this example?
4. Was patient safety at risk?

Box 5.1   The nursing student perspective—lessons learnt

Whether you are at university or in the clinical environment, there is much to learn, and students who have already navigated this path can provide excellent insights and strategies about everything from how to succeed in theory courses to what types of employment can assist you during your studies and how to secure that longed-for position after you graduate. The following are some tips from a high-achieving student to ensure success.

Tutorials and workshops

Tutorial and workshop sessions are often a fun and interactive way to learn the practical and theoretical content in the course. Most tutorial and workshop sessions are based on group work, and include scenarios that are based closely on the theoretical content. To get the most out of your tutorial or workshop:

- Come to the workshop or tutorial session prepared, having read the online content for that week or other required readings, and consider any questions that you may have to bring up during the tutorial.
- Engage in the scenarios and group work, as the practical application of your theoretical knowledge will help prepare you for clinical placements or your future employment.
- Discuss issues that arise with other students in the group—you will learn a great deal if you are open to the thoughts and viewpoints of others.

Workshop scenarios are very relevant to the types of circumstances that you may come across in your future employment. Engaging in these activities will allow you to understand how to deal with challenging circumstances and the types of problem-solving skills you may need in the workforce. The emphasis on teamwork mirrors the professional working environment, as health professionals continually work collaboratively in order to provide a high level of care.

Preparing for exams

Exam time can be very stressful, as there is often a great deal of theoretical content covered throughout a semester. In order to be adequately prepared for exams it is important to keep up to date with the theory content throughout the semester. Attempting to learn a semester's worth of work in a few short weeks is nearly impossible.

Towards the end of the semester there are often revision tutorials and lectures that summarise some of the topics that will be covered in the exam. While these lectures and tutorials will not cover everything you will need to know for the exam, they are a useful reminder of what to revisit over your revision period.

It is also sometimes possible to download your lectures, as PowerPoints or podcasts, from the online university resources, so that you can revise this material easily.

After revising a topic, it is often helpful to go over the material with other students in a study group, as you can ask each other questions and hopefully get a better understanding of the course content through these discussions.

Use the textbooks to look up any concepts that you are unsure of. Do not try to read the whole textbook and memorise large sections. Instead, try to achieve a good understanding of the material, and take notes. Refer to the text when clarifying or to obtain more information about particular topics.

Create your own practice questions and prepare answers for them; share these with other students.

Talk through questions and answers out loud to assist in remembering difficult concepts.

Clinical placements

Clinical placements are an essential part of the nursing degree. While they can be a daunting experience, they are also very rewarding. In order to make the most out of your clinical placement experience, it is important to ensure that you are adequately prepared.

- Consider what areas of nursing you are most interested in, as there are many different settings where you may have the opportunity to undertake your placement.
- Don't be afraid to choose a placement that may be outside your comfort zone, as this may be an area where you can learn a great deal and that will help you to decide if this may be an area of interest for employment in the future.
- Consider what types of skills you want to improve on throughout your placement. Consider your strengths and weaknesses, and use them to form the basis of possible learning objectives while on placement.
- Keep a journal of all your activities, as this can be used as further evidence to present to your facilitator or lecturer.
- Interact with the multidisciplinary team as much as possible—it is useful to have a good understanding of these services (for instance social work or physiotherapy) so that you can refer patients.

Take advantage of any opportunities to undertake tasks that you are not yet comfortable with, such as wound dressings or drain removal. Ask to first observe a registered nurse perform the task and, after reading the venue's policy and procedure manual, ask to perform the task under the supervision of the registered nurse. Once you have become comfortable with a particular task, it may be possible for you to demonstrate your accurate technique for other students while explaining the procedure. This will allow you to gain more experience and, additionally, will benefit other students' level of understanding.

Take note of the various roles undertaken by registered nurses within the clinical setting. Management, specialty areas and even education are often undertaken by registered nurses. If there is an area that you are particularly interested in, it may be possible for you to spend a short period of time with a registered nurse in that area, such as a mental health nurse or breast care nurse. Ask your facilitator if there is any possibility of something being arranged so that you can learn more about some of these specialised roles.

It is important to remember that while the clinical placement experience can be overwhelming, it is a learning environment. Allow yourself some time to settle into the clinical setting. Make the most of debriefing sessions organised by your clinical facilitator. Discuss any issues with some of your fellow students, as you may find that they are having similar issues or they may be able to provide solutions to problems you are facing.

Undergraduate employment opportunities

To maximise your learning opportunities and time within the clinical setting, a position within the field of nursing throughout your degree may be beneficial. Personal care attendant and assistant in nursing undergraduate positions are available in many acute care and aged care facilities. Within the acute care facilities undergraduate positions enable the student to undertake nursing duties under the indirect supervision of a registered nurse, depending on the venue's policies and procedures. This may include experience managing postoperative patients in consultation with a registered nurse, admissions and discharges, and preparing patients for theatre.

These employment positions can be beneficial to your future career, as your employment in the clinical setting is viewed positively by prospective employers. It is also likely that gaining employment in an acute setting may lead to a job prospect within this organisation, as the organisation will have gained insight into your work ethic and competence in a clinical environment.

Obtaining an assistant in nursing undergraduate position in an acute care setting provided us with valuable experience and insight into the role of the registered nurse. As our time management and organisational skills improved, so too did our confidence at practising in a more independent manner. It wasn't until we worked within this setting that we began to understand how the shift was structured, allowing patient care to be carried out in an orderly manner. We were also able to gain insight into the need for the registered nurse to be very flexible as, while a plan of action may be produced at the beginning of the shift, it may need to be rearranged to best manage the patients within your care. We were also able to observe that while there are standard practices within nursing, some tasks can be done in various ways while still following best practice and result in the same outcome for the patient. This enabled us to develop many problem-solving strategies.

Perhaps the most beneficial attribute from this position was the effective communication techniques that we gained in speaking with staff, patients and relatives. This has enabled us to gain further confidence, and we feel that we are now able to communicate effectively with staff and patients in a professional manner. This environment has also allowed us to develop our assessment skills.

This position allowed us to become very confident in some aspects of the job, which meant that we have now been able to focus our attention more on the responsibilities that are specific to the registered nurse role. This made clinical placements easier, because we had some knowledge of the manual handling and care roles, and were then able to focus more on complex procedures such as medication administration, wound care and IV therapy, and thus were offered more opportunities to practise these specialised skills.

Tips to survive the TPPP— Graduate nurse program

Transitioning from a student to a registered nurse and commencing your transition to professional practice program (TPPP) can be very daunting. Suddenly, you are responsible for the health and well-being of your patients without the close supervision that you received as a student. However, it is important to understand that this year will still provide you with a great deal of learning opportunities if you are able to make the most of them. As a newly registered nurse, you will still be developing your assessment and nursing skills and, as such, you will still require supervision from senior staff at various points in time. Even very experienced nurses will seek out the knowledge of other staff at times to ensure that their patient is receiving the care that they require. In order to make the most of your learning opportunities:

- Be aware of unfamiliar procedures in your area and request to assist or watch the RN perform these.
- Listen to handover of all of the ward patients and in your spare time read the case notes of any unusual diagnoses or discuss them with the nurse allocated to them.
- Research conditions or procedures with which you are not familiar.
- Discuss issues with the multidisciplinary team to gain an understanding of what different members can provide or assist with (for example, physiotherapy, social work). This will assist you to understand what the appropriate referrals are for various patients.
- Be respectful of other staff members, as you will be able to gain a great deal of knowledge from them.
- Be open to working in a team environment and accept help when it is offered— this is not a sign of weakness.

Use every experience as a learning opportunity. Inevitably, there will be some challenging cases and situations that are difficult to manage, or times when you do not have the support of your colleagues. However, through reflecting on these times you will have learnt valuable lessons and they will help to shape you as an experienced registered nurse.

SUMMARY

In this chapter we have looked at the processes of transition that students and new registered nurses go through in entering the clinical environment. Case studies and boxes provided in this chapter come from the experiences of new registered nurses who have been through the transition experience personally. Part-time work experience in healthcare, clinical placements and the formal TPPP were all discussed, as were experiences where nursing students move into the formal clinical environment for the first time. This chapter provided a more detailed overview of the TPPP, which you were introduced to in Chapter 1, and further explored your new responsibilities as a registered nurse. Embedded in this chapter is Benner's (2001) novice to expert model and, as you read through this chapter, you should begin to see how applicable this model is to your transition from student nurse to registered nurse.

Discussion questions

1. What are some key points you believe you will take with you from your student nurse experiences to your new role as a registered nurse?

2. From your perspective, how prepared are you to begin work as a registered nurse?

3. What are your expectations of the registered nurse role?

4. In your opinion, is it too soon to begin planning your career?

5. From your observations of nurses in advanced roles, such as clinical nurses and managers, what type of further study would you need to undertake and/or experience would you need to progress your career to this level?

Further Reading

Phillips, C, Esterman, A & Smith, C 2013, 'Predictors of successful transition to registered nurse', *Journal of Advanced Nursing*, vol. 69, issue 6, pp. 1314–22. This recent research study explored the impact of paid employment for nursing students on the transition into the registered nurse role.

Saintsing, D, Gibson, LM & Pennington, AW 2011, 'The novice nurse and clinical decision-making: how to avoid errors', *Journal of Nursing Management*, vol. 19, pp. 354–9. This article advises you how to avoid hospital errors.

Zerwekh, JA & Garneau, AZ 2012, *Nursing today: Transitions and trends*, 7th edn, Elsevier Saunders, St Louis Missouri. This is a useful text that discusses the process of transition for the new graduate registered nurse. While the context of this text book is American, the issues faced by the American graduate nurse are not dissimilar to the Australian graduate registered nurse.

Useful websites

Australian Government Workplace Health and Safety advice: http://australia.gov.au/topics/employment-and-workplace/ohs-workplace-health-and-safety.

Department of Health and Ageing Australian immunisation handbook: www.health.gov.au/internet/immunise/publishing.nsf/content/handbook-home.

Department of Health and Ageing Infection control guidelines: www.health.gov.au/internet/main/publishing.nsf/content/icg-guidelines-index.htm.

National Health and Medical Research Council's information on the regulation of health privacy in Australia: www.nhmrc.gov.au/guidelines/publications/nh53.

Workers Health Centre fact sheet on sleep and shift work: www.workershealth.com.au.

References

Alsup, S, Emerson, L, Lindell, A, Bechtle, M, & Whitmer, K 2006, 'Nursing cooperative partnership: a recruitment benefit', *Journal of Nursing Administration*, vol. 36, no. 4, pp. 163–6.

Australian Nursing and Midwifery Council & Australian College of Midwives 2006, *National competency standards for the midwife*, Australian Nursing and Midwifery Council, ACT.

Benner, P 2001, *From novice to expert: Excellence and power in clinical nursing practice*, Prentice-Hall, Upper Saddle River, NJ.

Berger, AM & Hobbs, BB 2005, 'Impact of shift work on the health and safety of nurses and patients', *Clinical Journal of Oncology Nursing*, vol. 10, no. 4, pp. 465–71.

Bradbury-Jones, C, Hughes, SM, Murphy, W, Parry, L & Sutton, J 2009, 'A new way of reflecting in nursing: the Peshkin approach', *Journal of Advanced Nursing*, vol. 65, no.11, pp. 2485–93.

Cope, P, Cuthbertson, P & Stoddart, B 2000, 'Situated learning in the practice placement', *Journal of Advanced Nursing*, vol. 31(4), pp. 850–6.

Department of Health and Ageing & National Health and Medical Research Council 2008, *Australian immunisation handbook*, 9th edn, Australian Government, Canberra, www .health.gov.au/internet/immunise/publishing.nsf/content/handbook-home, accessed 1 October 2011.

Elliott, M 2002, 'The clinical environment: a source of stress for undergraduate nurses', *Australian Journal of Advanced Nursing*, vol. 20, no. 1, pp. 34–8.

Kolb, DA, Boyatzis, R E, & Mainemelis, C 2000, 'Experiential learning theory: previous research and new directions', in *Perspectives on cognitive, learning, and thinking styles*, Sternberg & Zhang (eds), Lawrence Erlbaum, NJ.

Levett-Jones, T & Fitzgerald, M 2005, 'A review of graduate nurse transition programs in Australia', *Australian Journal of Advanced Nursing*, vol. 23, no. 2, pp. 40–5.

Levett-Jones T, Fahy K, Parsons K, & Mitchell A 2006, 'Enhancing nursing students' clinical placement experiences: a quality improvement project, *Contemporary Nurse*, vol. 23, no. 1: pp. 58–71 (doi: 10.5172/conu.2006.23.1.58).

Mayer, RM & Mayer, C 2000, 'Utilization-focused evaluation: evaluating the effectiveness of a hospital nursing orientation program', *Journal for Nurses in Staff Development*, vol. 16, no. 5, pp. 205–8.

Nursing and Midwifery Board of Australia 2013, *National competency standards for the registered nurse*, http://www.nursingmidwiferyboard.gov.au/Search. aspx?q=competency%20standards.

Pittet, D 2005, 'Infection control and quality health care in the new millennium', *Journal of Infection Control*, vol. 33, pp. 258–67.

Santuci, J 2004, 'Facilitating the transition into nursing practice', *Journal for Nurses in Staff Development*, vol. 20, no. 6, pp. 274–84.

Yonge, O, Myrick, F & Haase, M 2002, 'Student nurse stress in the preceptorship experience', *Nurse Educator*, vol. 27, no. 2, pp. 84–8.

Research in Clinical Practice

6

ANNE HOFMEYER

After reading this chapter, you will be able to:

- describe the role and significance of research in healthcare and nursing
- demonstrate a beginning understanding of research
- explain qualitative and quantitative approaches to research
- identify major elements of the research process
- describe the ethical considerations in healthcare research
- articulate the relevance of research knowledge for registered nurses
- discuss incorporating the forms of knowledge in clinical decision-making
- become a competent research consumer.

KEY TERMS

Critical appraisal
Evidence-based practice
Paradigm
Qualitative nursing research
Quantitative nursing research
Research

Introduction

The aim of this chapter is to introduce you to the key concepts of research and the importance of research in nursing and healthcare. Many undergraduate nursing students have a preconceived notion that understanding research and conducting research is difficult and confusing (Burrows & Baillie 1997), and 'is beyond them' (Ellis 2013, p. 1). Many report feeling stressed and anxious when having to enrol in research courses (Burrows & Baillie 1997). There is a lack of clarity about the relevance of research in everyday practice, how to source dependable evidence and how to use the evidence in clinical decision-making. So the focus of this chapter is to provide you with a basic understanding of the relevance of research, which we hope will allay anxieties that can act as a barrier to research use. Although few nurses will conduct original research (Gerrish & Lacey 2006), all registered nurses are expected to take responsibility to locate, critically appraise, understand and apply research findings in their current practice (Crookes & Davies 2004, p. xii).

It has long been considered that the hallmark of a profession is a research-based body of knowledge (ACN 2013; Hedges & Williams 2014; Greenwood 1957). The first nurse researcher was Florence Nightingale, who observed and investigated the environmental factors that affected the morbidity and mortality of soldiers injured in the Crimean war in the 1850s (ACN 2013). She reported her observations in her landmark publication, *Notes on nursing* (1859). Subsequently, the nursing literature contained little research until there was a marked increase in the 1950s in the United States, and then globally in the 1960s. Notably, the increase in research was associated with improvements in nurse education and doctoral programs for nurses (Polit & Beck 2008).

Recently, in Australia, various professional bodies have highlighted the foundational role of research in the practice and continuing professional development of registered nurses (Nursing and Midwifery Board of Australia 2006, Council of Deans of Nursing and Midwifery (ANZ) 2006). The Australian College of Nursing (2013) has developed a 'Nursing Research Position Statement' that clearly identifies the importance of research in improving nursing practice and health outcomes. The Nursing and Midwifery Board of Australia (2006) developed competency standards for the registered nurse, and have drawn clear links between research knowledge and use by registered nurses to ensure decision-making and practice within an evidence-based framework. Of specific note, we would like to draw your attention to the competency standards 3.1 to 3.4:

> *3.1 Identifies the relevance of research to improving individual/group health outcomes,*
> *3.2 Uses best available evidence, nursing expertise and respect for the values and beliefs of individuals/groups in the provision of nursing care,*
> *3.3 Demonstrates analytical skills in accessing and evaluating health information and research evidence,*
> *3.4 Supports and contributes to nursing and health care research (Nursing and Midwifery Board of Australia 2006, p. 4).*

Thus, this chapter will play a significant role in contributing to your beginning-level knowledge about research and will support your development in ways consistent with the challenge by Crookes and Davies (2004) discussed earlier and the expectation by the Nursing and Midwifery Board of Australia (2006). Specifically, Crookes and Davies (2004, p. xiii) propose the '4 *A*s of research' for consideration and attainment by nurses:

1. **A**wareness of and access to the research literature,
2. **A**ppreciation (or ability) to understand and critique the language of research,
3. **A**pplication of research findings to local practice settings, and
4. **A**bility to conduct original (primary) research independently or in a team.

So, although there is not an expectation that all nurses will undertake original research (the fourth *A*), it must be emphasised that all nurses are expected to demonstrate competence and application of relevant research knowledge in their practice (Daly et al. 2014 p. 140). However, a myriad of challenges and contextual factors exist in relation to using evidence in decision-making, so effective strategies are urgently required to address organisational and individual barriers, and to foster evidence-based practice. A key strategy for developing the necessary 'research literacy' is the provision of research education in undergraduate nursing programs (Halcomb & Peters 2009, p. 60). If students can be encouraged to appreciate the relevance of research education to practice, then it is more likely they will become 'evidence-based practitioners' (Halcomb & Peters 2009, p. 66), and value the importance of evidence-based nursing practice (Johnson et al. 2010; Blenkinsop 2003).

What is Research?

The basic purpose of **research** is to answer questions or solve problems of relevance in a systematic manner. Borbasi and Jackson (2012, p. 11) define research as 'a systematic process used to confirm and refine existing knowledge and to build new knowledge both inductively and deductively'. A **paradigm** is a 'world view that is based on a set of values and philosophical assumptions that are shared by a particular academic community and that guide their approach to research' (Schneider et al. 2013, p. 396). A paradigm also includes specific procedures and techniques that are coherent with the values and assumptions of the research community, and can be selected to investigate research questions and problems.

The traditional, positivist scientific paradigm is focused on items that can be tested, verified, counted and measured. Those researching in this quantitative paradigm investigate cause and effect. Data collection within the quantitative paradigm is deductive and strives for proof and objective reality. Deductive research begins with a hypothesis or theory about the effect of an intervention, and the researcher conducts the inquiry to confirm or reject, using deductive reasoning (Ellis 2013; Borbasi & Jackson 2012).

The naturalistic qualitative paradigm 'assumes that there are multiple interpretations of reality and that the goal of researchers working within this perspective is to understand how individuals construct their own reality within their social context' (Schneider et al. 2013, p. 395). The qualitative paradigm seeks to generate knowledge about how humans feel, think or understand their personal experiences (Ellis 2013). So knowledge is generated though inductive reasoning to uncover multiple new perspectives and subjective ways of knowing about a topic or

RESEARCH – A systematic process used to confirm and refine existing knowledge and to build new knowledge both inductively and deductively.

PARADIGM – A world view that is based on a set of values and philosophical assumptions that are shared by a particular academic community and that guide their approach to research.

ANNE HOFMEYER

human experience that is currently poorly understood or appreciated (Ellis 2013; Borbasi & Jackson 2012).

In order to become a knowledgeable consumer of research and develop your 'research literacy', it is essential to understand how research works and to become familiar with the key research terms. Entire textbooks are devoted to providing a comprehensive in-depth exposé of research; however, that aim is clearly beyond the scope of this short chapter. For that reason, you are encouraged to read widely and interrogate a variety of sources in your ongoing educational development in this topic. Review a glossary of common research terms that usually precedes the index in research textbooks as a starting point to learn about research terminology. Following are some terms that are useful to understand (Student Learning Centre 2012, p. 1):

- *Ethics (ethical) clearance:* when proposed research involves humans and/or animals, details of the research and how it will be conducted must be approved by an Ethics Approval committee. This process aims to protect the rights of humans and animals so that no harm occurs to either as a result of research.
- *Identifying a 'gap':* identifying a topic on which little or no research has been published, in order to come up with a useful, original study.
- *Reliability:* an instrument's ability to consistently and accurately measure the concept under study.
- *Representativeness (of a sample):* the degree to which a sample reflects the population from which it was drawn.
- *Rigour:* trustworthiness of documentation, procedures and ethics to establish credibility and transferability.
- *Theoretical framework:* theories which provide boundaries for the study and guide all stages.
- *Validity:* the ability of an instrument to measure what it is supposed to measure'.

As illustrated in table 6.1, within each research paradigm are methodological approaches that provide the coherent structure to conduct the research.

As illustrated in table 6.1, the methods utilised to collect data need to be consistent with the research paradigm and methodology which provides a framework for conducting the study.

What is evidence and EBP?

EVIDENCE-BASED PRACTICE (EBP) – The use of the best clinical evidence in making patient care decisions, and such evidence typically comes from research conducted by nurses and other healthcare professionals.

Global debates continue about the nature of **evidence-based practice**, and the barriers and incentives to improve clinical decision-making. Debates about what constitutes 'evidence' and its relevance to clinical practice by nurses continues among researchers, clinicians, educators and policy-makers (Sackett et al. 2000; Laschinger et al. 1990). A physician called Archie Cochrane coined the term

TABLE 6.1 EXPLANATION OF THE RESEARCH PARADIGMS

	POSITIVIST PARADIGM QUANTITATIVE	INTERPRETIVE PARADIGM QUALITATIVE	CRITICAL PARADIGM
Philosophical Position	Empirico-analytical Reductionist level Search for truth Objective reality Controlled Deductive reasoning Subjects	Naturalistic Post-modern Holistic level Search for meaning Inductive reasoning Participants	Post-modern Post-structural Emancipatory Holistic level Search for meaning Inductive reasoning Participants
Methodology	Randomised controlled trial Cohort study Case-control studies Cross-sectional studies	Phenomenology Grounded theory Ethnography Case study	Feminist research Action research Critical ethnology
Data collection	Surveys Questionnaires Experiments } numbers	Observation Interviews Focus groups } words	Observation Interviews Focus groups
Researcher position	Distant	Interactive approach Immersed in the setting	Interactive approach Immersed in the setting

Adapted from Schneider et al. (2013, pp. 25–6).

'evidence-based practice' in the early 1970s (Sackett 1996) so the evidence-based practice (EBP) movement emerged as a means of improving clinical practice through the use of current evidence. Evidence-based practice (EBP) is defined as 'the use of the best clinical evidence in making patient care decisions and such evidence typically comes from research conducted by nurses and other health care professionals' (Polit & Beck 2008, p. 3). Dawes et al. (2005, p. 4) state that EBP 'aims to provide the best possible evidence at the point of clinical (or management) contact'. With that definition in mind, Richardson-Tench et al. (2011, p. 12) propose the following relevant questions:

- What is the best possible evidence?
- Who judges it?
- How?

- Why?
- For whom?
- Under what circumstances?

Empirical evidence that results from quantitative studies (specifically randomised control trials (RCT)) was initially considered the 'gold standard' for EBP (Schneider et al. 2013).

The National Health and Medical Research Council (NHMRC) in Australia provides a guide about the levels of evidence (hierarchy) preferred for developing EBP clinical practice guidelines (NHMRC 2009). Notably, evidence generated from quantitative research methods is considered the best type of evidence (Richardson-Tench et al. 2011). The following hierarchy of evidence shown in table 6.2 is based on summaries from the National Health and Medical Research Council (2009), the Oxford Centre for Evidence-based Medicine Levels of Evidence (2011) and Melynk and Fineout-Overholt (2011).

The exclusion of qualitative research findings as evidence in EBP has attracted criticism (Richardson-Tench et al. 2011). Daly et al (2007, p. 45) offer four levels of hierarchy for assessing the contribution of qualitative research studies of evidence for practice, as shown in table 6.3.

TABLE 6.2 HIERARCHY OF EVIDENCE

Level 1	Systematic review of all relevant randomised controlled trials
Level 11	At least one well-designed randomised controlled trial
Level 111	Evidence obtained from well-designed controlled trials without randomisation
Level 1V	Well-designed cohort studies, case control studies, interrupted time series with a control group, historically controlled studies, interrupted time series without a control group or with case- series
Level V	Systematic reviews of descriptive and qualitative studies
Level V1	Single descriptive and qualitative studies
Level V11	Expert opinion from clinicians, authorities and/or reports of expert committees or based on physiology

TABLE 6.3 HIERARCHY OF EVIDENCE-FOR-PRACTICE IN QUALITATIVE RESEARCH

Level 1	Generalisable studies
Level 11	Conceptual studies
Level 111	Descriptive studies
Level 1V	Single case study

Daly et al. (2007, p. 43) assert that this hierarchy of evidence-for-practice specific to qualitative methods offers researchers a useful guide to assess the quality of the studies and evidence to utilise in clinical practice.

Four forms of knowledge

It is now more widely accepted that evidence or knowledge can be derived from many sources. We are reminded that patient-centred care incorporates the knowledge and preferences of the patient in decision-making. So evidence-based practice is now proposed by Rycroft-Malone et al. (2004) as an approach to decision-making that integrates the best available evidence and knowledge with clinical expertise and patient values and preferences. Communication and respect are critical features of this approach to deliver safe and quality health care. Therefore, evidence derived from qualitative research is now incorporated in EBP (Schneider et al. 2013). This broader view of which sources of knowledge constitute dependable evidence for clinical decision argues for the inclusion of sources other than research (Schneider et al. 2013; Rycroft-Malone et al. 2004). To explain this view, Rycroft-Malone et al. (2004) differentiate between 'propositional' generalisable knowledge derived from research and 'non-propositional' knowledge that arises in practice from nurses, patients and families, and is specific to the local contexts. Rycroft-Malone et al. (2004, p. 81) discuss 'the potential contribution of four types of evidence in the delivery of care; namely, research, clinical experience, patient experience and information from the local context'. The authors challenge nurses to incorporate several sources of knowledge in their clinical decision-making when planning quality care with their patients and their families.

What is nursing research?

The Australian College of Nursing (2013 p. 1) defines **nursing research** as 'scientific inquiry (qualitative and quantitative) designed to develop knowledge about health and well-being. It is essential for the nursing profession to strengthen its research culture and support evidence-based nursing practice, to optimise the health and well-being of people and society.' The ACN (2013 p. 2) recommends that 'nursing research is integrated into all undergraduate and postgraduate nursing courses to (i) build research capacity, (ii) promote the role of and contribution of nurses to evidence-based practice, and (iii) engender that understanding of the critical role of research in practice development'.

It is therefore essential that nurse educators demystify the topic of research and respond to students' anxieties through innovative teaching about the relevance of evidence to practice, and motivate students' to engage with and become consumers of research.

NURSING RESEARCH – Scientific inquiry (qualitative and quantitative) designed to develop knowledge about health and well-being. It is essential for the nursing profession to strengthen its research culture and support evidence-based nursing practice, to optimise the health and well-being of people and society.

ANNE HOFMEYER

The research process

The research process is a standard process that includes all elements found in a research proposal and reported in a publication. The stages of the research process can be understood in terms of the following coherent steps (Ellis 2013; Blenkinsop 2003); namely:

- Identify an issue or problem in need of research, formulate a researchable idea.
- Conduct a literature review, read relevant literature, identify a gap.
- State the purpose of the research.
- Identify the research questions, aims, objectives or hypotheses.
- Design the study.
- Collect the data.
- Analyse the data.
- Interpret and discuss findings in the context of the literature.
- Evaluate, report and disseminate the findings.

Critical reflection

The identification of a research topic usually occurs in response to a problem that arises in clinical practice. Reflect on experiences you had in your previous clinical learning placements during your undergraduate program.

- Make a list of problems or gaps in the knowledge that arose during your placement.
- How did the problem or lack of knowledge about an element of nursing care affect the quality care of patients?
- What evidence or knowledge was missing?
- What strategies were used by you and the registered nurses to address the problem or knowledge gap?
- How could you think and act differently about the problem now?
- Make a list of questions related to the problem that you would like to investigate.

Locating research

Sources of EBP information can be found in bibliographic databases such as Medline, CINAHL, PsychINFO, Embase, DARE, Cochrane Library, the Australian Digital Thesis Program and Conference Papers Index, to name a few. Nurses are required to demonstrate competence in locating relevant and dependable knowledge through a range of sources. Therefore, it is essential to invest time in becoming familiar with the wide range of electronic and print databases, websites and other resources available in your local library. There is a wealth of information available online and librarians provide a range of specific training courses to build capacity and literacy. Working collaboratively with librarians is a wise strategy for students and nurses to improve their success in effective database searching, generating key words, and the Medical Subject Headings MeSH terms for specific online searching in the various bibliographic databases. MeSH is a terminology used to index journal articles and books in the life sciences and the terms can be used to facilitate searching.

Literature sources fall into two categories: primary sources and secondary sources. Primary sources is the term used to describe scholarly original research and theoretical literature that are published in the form of refereed journal articles, books, monographs and academic higher degree postgraduate theses (Schneider et al. 2013). Secondary sources are usually summaries or critiques of primary review papers and research studies, where you are not reading the original work, but what the author considers are the main points and interpretations. So a guide here is to ascertain the credibility of the author writing the secondary source and whether the work has been published in a refereed journal or in a credible resource that promotes EBP. Some examples of credible resources (i.e. journals, organisations and clearing houses) that have used secondary sources to develop clinical practice guidelines that support evidence-based practice are listed at the end of the chapter in the Useful websites section. This is not an exhaustive list, so you can add to this list as you build your knowledge in this area.

Developing research questions

There is a perception that developing a research question is a simple process. But this stage in the research process is crucial to ensure rigour, clarity about the research aim and focus, the parameters, and the knowledge to be generated. Questions typically serve one of two purposes, either to identify the current evidence (literature) about a topic or to address a gap in the literature where is there scant evidence (Ellis 2013). It is necessary to clearly define your search by setting parameters about the year to limit the search (Schneider et al. 2013) and use of Boolean operators that act as joining words (i.e. or, and, near, not) when conducting the search in the relevant databases (Borbasi & Jackson 2012).

Mantzoukas (2008, p. 375) contends that a 'good qualitative research question requires to be structured in such a manner as to successfully convey sufficient information about the topic of the study, the participants of the study, the context of the study, the time of the study and the way the study will be conducted'. There needs to be coherence between the 'philosophical/theoretical propositions of the qualitative paradigms' and the manner in which the researcher intends to structure and conduct the study (Mantzoukas 2008, p. 376). Specifically, 'the structure needs to adequately answer the who, when, where, what, how and why of the study'

(Mantzoukas 2008, p. 376). An example of a qualitative question that features the outlined structure is: 'Understanding through interpretative phenomenology (how) students' (who) experiences in completing a portfolio as a formal assessment method (what) for a contemporary (when) university course in the UK (where)' (Mantzoukas 2008, p. 376).

There are commonly accepted models to formulate research questions and plan how to search the bibliographic databases. Models are typically referred to by an acronym that guides the development of the research question in a logical and systematic manner.

The SPICE model can be used to frame and generate a qualitative research question or area of inquiry (Ellis 2013). SPICE refers to:

- Setting
- Perspective
- Intervention
- Comparison
- Evaluation.

Critical reflection

Using the SPICE model, plan how you could generate a researchable question to investigate a problem that you identified in the previous critical reflection box.
- Write down the question.
- Decide if the problem is better addressed using a quantitative or a qualitative approach.
- Discuss your rationale.

The PICO/T model can be used to help frame clinical questions for research studies and also identifies keywords that can guide the literature search (Ellis 2013; Schneider et al. 2013). This process helps define the search by establishing parameters and helps to identify relevant literature. The PICO/T model is applicable to research studies that include an intervention. The acronym stands for:

- Patient or problem
- Intervention of interest
- Comparison
- Outcome
- Timeframe (not always used, Schneider et al. 2013).

For example, the *patient* could refer to patients in an outpatient department with diabetes. The *intervention* could be the education program. *Comparison* could be the knowledge of the patients before and following the education program, and the *outcome* could refer to the improvement in the patients' self-management of diabetes. So the research question could be to investigate the effect of an education program on a patient's understanding of managing their diabetes.

Critical reflection

Using the PICO/T model, plan how you could generate a researchable question to investigate a problem that you identified in the previous critical reflection box.
- Write down the question.
- Decide if the problem is better addressed using a quantitative or a qualitative approach.
- Discuss your rationale.

There is now wide use of the reliable PICO/T search strategy to formulate questions and in conducting systematic reviews of quantitative research (Cooke et al. 2012). However, there are limitations. Cooke et al. (2012, p. 1436) note that the 'PICO tool is not an optimal working strategy for qualitative evidence synthesis'. The authors promote SPIDER an alternative search strategy tool for qualitative/ mixed methods research:
- Sample
- Phenomenon of interest
- Design
- Evaluation
- Research type.

The development of the research question is a crucial step in the design of the research study. These models are offered as a guide to clarify thinking and formulate a sound framework that will generate new, useful evidence to solve clinical problems. Further reading about the models is indicated to foster your competence in this step in the research process.

Critiquing the evidence

Undergraduate nursing students are expected to generate researchable problems, conduct literature searches to identify credible studies, critique the evidence, and use relevant findings in clinical decision-making, thus building their 'research literacy'. A strategy for success is to become familiar with robust critique tools to appraise the methodological quality quantitative and qualitative research articles. It is important to read and re-read studies, and clarify unfamiliar terms in the glossary of a research textbook. The research article is usually set out in the following sections:

- *Abstract:* that provides a summary of the purpose of the study, methods, participants, results and conclusions. It is either structured or as one paragraph.
- *Introduction:* introduces the issue or problem, purpose of the research study and the research question.
- *Background/literature review:* establishes context for the study, the significance of the issue, and identifies what is known and not known (the gap in knowledge).
- *Methods:* outlines the study design, who participated, where they were located, and how the data was collected and analysed.
- *Findings/results:* provides a summary of the significant outcomes of the study.
- *Discussion:* discusses the implications of the research outcomes in relation to the research question and compares and contrasts to the existing literature. Identifies how the findings/results may have contributed to addressing the gap in the knowledge.
- *Conclusions:* presents a summary of the significant points in the study, proposes recommendations and possible directions for future research.
- *Reference list:* contains all the sources that were cited in the article.

Critical appraisal is 'the process of systematically examining research evidence to assess its validity, results and relevance before using it to inform a decision' (Hill & Spittlehouse 2003). Critical appraisal is an integral process in evidence-based practice. Critical appraisal aims to identify methodological flaws in the literature and provide the reader with a rigorous framework to make informed decisions about the quality of research evidence. There are numerous critical appraisal tools available to guide the evaluation of published quantitative and qualitative research literature. See, for example, the list of critical appraisal tools on the International Centre for Allied Health Evidence (ICAHE) that can be selected to guide the critique and critical appraisal of the following research evidence:

- Randomised controlled trials
- Non-randomised controlled trials
- Other quantitative research
- Case studies
- Qualitative research
- Mixed methods research
- Systematic reviews
- Meta-analysis
- Outcome measures.

CRITICAL APPRAISAL – The 'process of systematically examining research evidence to assess its validity, results and relevance before using it to inform a decision' (Hill & Spittlehouse 2003).

A framework developed by Caldwell et al. (2011, p. e3) for nursing students, addresses both the quantitative and qualitative research critical appraisal process using the following series of questions:

- *'Does the title reflect the content? The title should be informative and indicate the focus of the study. It should allow the reader to easily interpret the content of the study. An inaccurate or misleading title can confuse the reader.*
- *Are the authors credible? Researchers should hold appropriate academic qualifications and be linked to a professional field relevant to the research.*
- *Does the abstract summarize the key components? The abstract should provide a short summary of the study. It should include the aim of the study, outline of the methodology and the main findings. The purpose of the abstract is to allow the reader to decide if the study is of interest to them.*
- *Is the rationale for undertaking the research clearly outlined? The author should present a clear rationale for the research, setting it in context of any current issues and knowledge of the topic to date.*
- *Is the literature review comprehensive and up-to-date? The literature review should reflect the current state of knowledge relevant to the study and identify any gaps or conflicts. It should include key or classic studies on the topic as well as up to date literature. There should be a balance of primary and secondary sources.*
- *Is the aim of the research clearly stated? The aim of the study should be clearly stated and should convey what the researcher is setting out to achieve.*
- *Are all ethical issues identified and addressed? Ethical issues pertinent to the study should be discussed. The researcher should identify how the rights of informants have been protected and informed consent obtained. If the research is conducted within the NHS then there should be indication of Local Research Ethics committee approval.*
- *Is the methodology identified and justified? The researcher should make clear which research strategy they are adopting, i.e. qualitative or quantitative. A clear rationale for the choice should also be provided, so that the reader can judge whether the chosen strategy is appropriate for the study. At this point the student is asked to look specifically at the questions that apply to the paradigm appropriate to the study they are critiquing (Table 2). To complete their critique, the final questions students need to address are applied to both quantitative and qualitative studies.*
- *Are the results presented in a way that is appropriate and clear? Presentation of data should be clear, easily interpreted and consistent.*
- *Is the discussion comprehensive? In quantitative studies the results and discussion are presented separately. In qualitative studies these maybe integrated. Whatever the mode of presentation, the researcher should compare and contrast the findings with that of previous research on the topic. The discussion should be balanced and avoid subjectivity.*
- *Is the conclusion comprehensive? Conclusions must be supported by the findings. The researcher should identify any limitations to the study. There may also be*

*recommendations for further research, or if appropriate, implications for practice
in the relevant field'.*

(Caldwell et al. 2011, p. e3).

Critical appraisal tools provide a series of questions to guide the critique of a research article. It is important to ensure that the tool/s you use are appropriate for their purpose and the type of study you plan to appraise and evaluate. The questions help you assess the quality of the research conducted and the rigour (robustness) and trustworthiness of the results. You are then primed to make judgments about the applicability and usefulness of the results in your clinical decision-making, to provide quality evidence-based care for patients.

Ethical considerations

All research must be conducted in accordance with the strict guidelines that govern the conduct of researchers and the manner in which research is conducted (National Health and Medical Research Council 2007), and review and approval must be gained from institutional human research ethics committees (HRECs). All researchers are required to undergo training about the ethical guidelines and requirements for conducting research according to the NHMRC and HREC. Guidelines specify the storing of data, obtaining informed consent, ensuring confidentiality and anonymity, and reporting of research findings. The National Statement (2007, p. 3) advises that 'all human interaction, including the interaction involved in human research, has ethical dimensions. However, 'ethical conduct' is more than simply doing the right thing. It involves acting in the right spirit out of an abiding respect and concern for one's fellow creatures. The National Statement on 'Ethical Conduct in Human Research' is therefore oriented to something more fundamental than ethical 'dos' and 'don'ts'; namely, an ethos that should permeate the way those engaged in human research approach all that they do in their research'.

There are two aspects to be considered in the management of research data: the accurate reporting of data, and the 'physical management' and storage of research data (Chater 2011, pp. 69). Health Research Ethics Committees (HREC) require researchers to provide specific details about where all data will be stored, in what formats (electronic and paper), security measures undertaken (such as stored on a password-protected computer or in a locked filing cabinet), who will have access to the data, and the length of time that the data will be stored. When individuals consent to participate they are assured of privacy, anonymity and confidentiality with regard to their identity and any data collected from them. Increasing emphasis has been directed to the use, security and storage of USB flash drives, digital recorders and laptops that contain research data. This is due to the rising incidence of such items being reported lost or misplaced. The physical management of confidential data also includes security measures taken when using computer software packages such as SPSS Statistics, used for quantitative statistical analysis, and NVivo for qualitative data analysis.

THEORY TO PRACTICE

Hannah is a registered nurse who has recently graduated with a Bachelor of Nursing and is now working in a large emergency department setting. She is interested in the attendance of many people with minor or non-urgent illnesses and wonders why they believe it is better to attend the emergency department rather than visiting the local general practice clinic. The general practice clinic is open 7 days a week from 7am to 10pm and no appointment is necessary. Hannah drives past the general practice clinic on her way to work and often notices the waiting area is empty.

The impact on extended waiting times and general flow-through of patients in the emergency department is creating significant safety problems for other patients with more severe morbidities and increasing the pressure on nursing staff. The extended waiting times have resulted in poor care experiences for a number of older patients and aggressive reactions from others. Sick leave has increased in recent weeks and float nurses are rejecting relief shifts in the emergency department.

You are the clinical manager in the emergency department. Hannah has asked for your help to plan how to investigate this clinical problem. What would you advise Hannah in relation to the following stages in the research process:

- Designing a researchable question
- Developing a search strategy
- Locating relevant literature
- Critiquing the literature effectively
- Extracting relevant information and writing a literature review
- Selecting a qualitative or quantitative approach to investigate the research problem
- Identifying the sample/participants
- Mode of data collection
- Approaching and including other nurses in the research process.

Discussion Questions

Provide approximately four discussion questions.

1. What do you think would be the organisational barriers to change?
2. What do you think would the barriers at the unit level need to change in order to improve this situation?
3. What forms of knowledge would you need to include in this decision-making process and how would you go about it?
4. How would you plan to collaborate with the nursing staff at the general practice clinic?
5. What would need to be implemented to achieve sustainable outcomes and long-term change to improve this current situation?

ANNE HOFMEYER

SUMMARY

Nursing students and registered nurses have a responsibility to participate in stages of the research process appropriate to their educational development. They must develop a basic understanding of research to fulfil their professional competencies and collaborate with other professionals, patients and their families in evidence-based decision-making to provide quality health care. Learning about the process of research and key terms is a key strategy to change perceptions and appreciate the relevance of research knowledge so all nurses become competent consumers of research evidence-to-practice.

All nurses must develop critical appraisal skills to evaluate research studies and engage in continuous educational development to improve their practice. There are many critical appraisal tools that provide a series of questions to guide critique of the research literature. It is important to ensure that the tools selected are appropriate for their purpose and the type of research to evaluate.

Discussion questions

1. Poor utilisation (application/implementation) of research knowledge in clinical decision-making continues to be a feature in nursing. List three elements that you consider could act as barriers to using research evidence in your clinical practice.

2. What do you think is the most important reason you should use current research evidence in your clinical practice? Provide a justification for your answer.

3. An initial step in becoming a knowledge research consumer involves understanding the language of research. How would you explain the different paradigms to another nurse and why it is important to understand the components of each?

4. Registered nurses should seek out opportunities to participate in research so they can learn aspects of the research process. What social and organisational elements support opportunities to participate?

5. Think about a patient that you provided care for during a previous clinical placement. Describe the patient and their social situation and relationships. Discuss how you would go about incorporating several sources of knowledge in your clinical decision-making when planning quality patient-centred care with that patient and their family.

Further Reading

Caldwell, K, Henshaw, L & Taylor, G 2011, 'Developing a framework for critiquing health research: an early evaluation', *Nurse Education Today*, vol. 31, no. 8, pp. e1–7.

Kaplan, L 2012, 'Reading and critiquing a research article', *American Nurse Today*, vol. 7, no. 10, http://www.americannursetoday.com accessed 17 February 2014.

National Health and Medical Research Council 2009, *NHMRC levels of evidence and grades for recommendations for developers of guidelines*, Australian Government: National Health and Medical Research Council.

Useful websites

As a resource to evidence-based practice, follow the links to lesson one of the introductory tutorials from the University of Minnesota (http://evidence.ahc.umn.edu/ebn.htm). This tutorial provides a detailed description of the evidence-based practice process.

Joanna Briggs Institute (JBI)(http://www.joannabriggs.org) provides a range of resources such as Best Practice Information Sheets, JBI Systematic Reviews and Evaluation Cycle Reports. Take particular note of the evidence-based model used by JBI in the left-hand column. Many health care organisations have membership with JBI so health professionals can access dependable evidence to inform clinical decision-making.

National Institute of Clinical Studies (NICS) (http://www.nhmrc.gov.au/nics/index.htm) is part of the National Health and Medical Research Council (NHMRC) and provides fact sheets about the best available evidence to improve health care. When reviewing this website take particular notice of the following: NICS Overview fact sheet and the NICS Programs overview fact sheet.

The Cochrane Library (http://www.thecochranelibrary.com/view/0/index.html) provides access to several main databases including The Cochrane Database of Systematic Reviews. Cochrane systematic reviews are ranked as the highest level of research evidence (Level One) as the systematic reviews are undertaken using the NHMRC criteria. At first glance, it probably looks very complicated, so start with the User Guide: User Guide to the Cochrane Library http://www.nicsl.com.au/cochrane/guide. asp(http://www.cochrane.org.au/libraryguide/guide.php) then review The Cochrane Library Databases and Finding information in the Cochrane Library (http://www. cochrane.org.au/libraryguide/guide_data.php)

Best-practice information sheets are resources that provide clear and concise information for clinician and recommend the best available evidence for clinical practice. They include information about the types of research evidence available on the topic including studies reviewed and evidence based recommendations about the topic.

The McMaster University School of Nursing in Ontario, Canada has links on the website to a number of repositories of dependable knowledge such as the National Collaborating Centre for Methods and Tools at www.nccmt.ca

Journals

Journal of Clinical Nursing; Evidence Based Nursing; Implementation Science; Worldviews on Evidence-Based Nursing.

Organisations

Cochrane Collaboration. http://www.cochrane.org.

Excellence in Research Australia. http://www.arc.gov.au/era/default.htm.

National Institute of Clinical Guidelines. http://www.clinicalguidelines.gov.au.

New Zealand Guidelines Group. http://www.nzgg.org.nz/.

Critical appraisal

McMaster University. Centre for Evidence-Based Medicine (CEBM) http://fhswedge.csu. mcmaster.ca/cepftp/qasite/CriticalAppraisal.html.

International Center for Allied Health Evidence. http://www.unisa.edu.au/Research/Sansom-Institute-for-Health-Research/Research-at-the-Sansom/Research-Concentrations/Allied-Health-Evidence/Resources/CAT/.

References

American Nurses' Association Commission on Nursing Research 1981, 'Guidelines for the investigative functions of nurses', ANA, Kansas City, Missouri.

Australian College of Nursing 2013, 'Nursing research position statement', ACN Ltd Canberra, http://www.acn.edu.au, accessed 5 February 2014.

Blenkinsop, C 2003, 'Research: an essential skill of a graduate nurse?' *Nurse Education Today*, vol. 23, no. 2, pp. 83–8.

Borbasi, S & Jackson, D 2012, *Navigating the maze of research*, 3rd edn, Mosby Elsevier, Chatswood NSW.

Burrows, DE, & Baillie, L 1997, 'A strategy for teaching research to adult branch diploma students', *Nurse Education Today*, vol. 17, no. 1, pp. 39–45.

Caldwell, K, Henshaw, L & Taylor, G 2011 'Developing a framework for critiquing health research: an early evaluation', *Nurse Education Today*, vol. 31, no. 8, pp. e1–7.

Chater, K 2011 'Ethical and legal considerations in research', in S Jirojwong, M Johnson & A Welch (eds), *Research methods in nursing & midwifery: pathways to evidence-based practice*, Oxford University Press, South Melbourne, Victoria, pp. 62–86.

Cooke, A, Smith, D & Booth, A 2012, 'Beyond PICO: the SPIDER tool for qualitative evidence synthesis', *Qualitative Health Research*, vol. 22, no. 10, pp. 1435–43.

Council of Deans of Nursing and Midwifery (ANZ) n.d. www.cdnm.edu.au accessed 5 February 2014.

Crookes, P & Davies, S (eds) 2004, *Research into practice: essential skills for reading and applying research in nursing and health care*, Baillière Tindall, Edinburgh.

Daly, J, Elliott, D, Chang, E & Usher, E 2014, 'Research in nursing: concepts and processes', in J Daly, S Speedy & D Jackson (eds), *Contexts of nursing*, 4th edn, Elsevier, Sydney, pp. 137–56.

Daly, J, Willis, K, Small, R, Green, J, Welch, N, Kealy, M & Hughes, E 2007, 'A hierarchy of evidence for assessing qualitative health research', *Journal of Clinical Epidemiology*, vol. 60, no. 1, pp. 43-9.

Dawes, M, Davies, P, Gray, A, Mant, J, Seers, K & Snowball, R 2005, *Evidence-based practice: a primer for health care professionals*, 2nd edn, Elsevier Churchill Livingstone, Edinburgh.

Ellis, P 2013, *Understanding research for nursing students*, 2nd edn, Sage Learning Matters, UK.

Gerrish, K & Lacey, A (eds) 2006, *The research process in nursing*, 5th edn, Blackwell Publishing Ltd., Oxford.

Greenwood, E 1957, 'Attributes of a profession' *Social Work* vol. 2, no. 3, pp. 45–55.

Halcomb, EJ & Peters, K 2009, 'Nursing student feedback on undergraduate research education: implications for teaching and learning,' *Contemporary Nurse*, vol. 33, no. 1, pp. 59–68.

Hedges, C & Williams, B 2014, *Anatomy of research for nurses*, Sigma Theta Tau International; Indianapolis, Indiana USA.

Hill, A & Spittlehouse, C 2003, 'What is critical appraisal?,' *Evidence-Based Medicine*, vol. 3, no. 2, pp. 1–8.

Johnson, N, List-Ivankovic, J, Eboh, WO, Ireland, J, Adams, D, Mowatt, E & Martindale, S 2010, 'Research and evidence based practice: using a blended approach to teaching and learning in undergraduate nurse education,' *Nurse Education in Practice*, vol. 10, no. 1, pp. 43–7.

Laschinger, HS, Johnson, G & Kohr, R 1990, 'Building undergraduate nursing students' knowledge of the research process in nursing,' *Journal of Nursing Education*, vol. 29, no. 3, pp. 114–17.

Mantzoukas, S 2008, 'Facilitating research students in formulating qualitative research questions,' *Nurse Education Today*, vol. 28, no. 3, pp. 371–7.

Melynyk, B & Fineout-Overholt, E 2011, *Evidence-based practice in nursing & healthcare: a guide to best practice*, 2nd edn, Wolters Kluwer, Lippincott Williams & Wilkins, Philadelphia.

National Health and Medical Research Council 2009, *NHMRC levels of evidence and grades for recommendations for developers of guidelines*, Australian Government: NHMRC.

National Statement on Ethical Conduct in Human Research 2007, National Health and Medical Research Council, Australian Government http://www.nhmrc.gov.au/_files_nhmrc/publications/attachments/e72_national_statement_130207.pdf accessed16 February 2014.

Nursing and Midwifery Board of Australia 2006, *National competency standards for the registered nurse*, Nursing and Midwifery Board of Australia, Victoria, http://www.nursingmidwiferyboard.gov.au/Codes-Guidelines-Statements/Codes-Guidelines.aspx, accessed 5 February 2014.

OCEBM Levels of Evidence Working Group Oxford 2011, *The Oxford 2011 Levels of Evidence*, Oxford Centre for Evidence-Based Medicine http://www.cebm.net/index.aspx?o=1025 accessed 5 February 2014.

Polit, DF & Beck, CT 2008, *Nursing research: generating and assessing evidence for nursing practice*, 8th edn, Lippincott Williams & Wilkins, Philadelphia, USA.

Richardson-Tench, M, Taylor, B, Kermode, S & Roberts, K 2011, *Research in nursing: evidence for best practice*, 4th edn, Cengage Learning Australia Pty Limited, South Melbourne, Victoria.

Rycroft-Malone, J, Seer, K, Titchen, A, Harvey, G, Kitson, A & McCormack, B 2004, 'What counts as evidence in evidence-based practice?', *Journal of Advanced Nursing*, vol. 47, no. 1, pp. 81–90.

Schneider, Z, Whitehead, D, Lo-Biondo-Wood, G & Haber, J 2013, *Nursing and midwifery research: methods and appraisal for evidence-based practice*, 4th edn, Mosby Elsevier, Chatswood NSW, Australia.

Sackett, D & Rosenberg, W 1995, 'The need for evidence-based medicine', *Journal of the Royal Society Medicine*, vol. 88, no. 11, pp. 620–4.

Sackett, D (1996) 'Evidence-based medicine: what it is and what it isn't', *British Medical Journal*, vol. 312, no. 7023, pp. 71–2.

Sackett, DL, Straus, SE, Richardson, WS, Rosenberg, W & Haynes, RB 2000, *Evidence-based medicine: how to practice and teach EBM*, Churchill Livingstone, Edinburgh.

Student Learning Centre 2012, *Critiquing research articles*, Flinders University, Adelaide, pp. 1–4. http://www.flinders.edu.au accessed 4 February 2014.

Australia's Healthcare System

7

MARIA FEDORUK AND LUISA TOFFOLI

LEARNING OBJECTIVES

After reading this chapter, you will be able to:

- describe Australia's healthcare system
- describe the healthcare workforce in Australia
- discuss the issues facing the nursing workforce in Australia
- describe the healthcare system you work in.

KEY TERMS

eHealth
Functional flexibility
Health literacy
mHealth
National Health Agreement (NHA)
Numerical flexibility
Professional skills escalation
Work–life balance

Australia's Healthcare System

As a registered nurse, you should have an understanding of how Australia's healthcare system works. This is how Duckett and Willcox (2011, p. 1) summarise Australia's healthcare system:

- Healthcare is a system involving inputs (finance, workforce), processes, outputs and outcomes. It is situated in the broader socio-political environment which it both is affected by and affects.
- The outputs and outcomes of the health care system include individual or person-level outputs (patients treated), and outcomes (improved quality of life) and wider outputs/outcomes (research outputs, strong communities, changed environments). Health outputs and health outcomes are not always distributed evenly across all members of a society.
- The health care system can be evaluated in terms of its impact on equity, quality, acceptability and efficiency.
- The organisation and design of health systems must have regard to the differences between the need, demand and supply of health services. The 'need' for health services is not objective but is framed within a social and political context.

A visual representation of Australia's healthcare system is provided in figure 7.1. It shows you healthcare from a systems perspective. All organisations have inputs, processes and outputs or outcomes. Underpinning any set of inputs is the ability to pay for these inputs. Financing is critical to obtaining inputs such as workforce, capital, information and communication technologies, and supplies (Duckett & Willcox 2011). Thus, the availability of financial resources drives clinical and non-clinical decision-making in healthcare organisations.

FIGURE 7.1 ANALYSIS FRAMEWORK OF AUSTRALIA'S HEALTHCARE SYSTEM

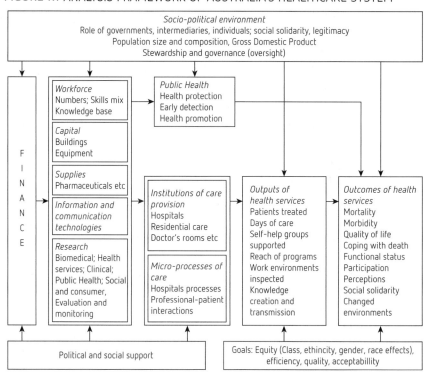

Source: S Duckett & S Willcox 2011, *The Australian health care system*, 4th edn, Oxford University Press, Melbourne, p. 3.2.

The Commonwealth government, through the Department of Health, devolves the management of Australia's healthcare system to each state and territory government. You are encouraged to familiarise yourself with the resources located within the Commonwealth, state and territory government websites relating to Australia's healthcare system, as this will help inform your practice, alerting you to new health policy initiatives that may result in new health treatments or models of service delivery.

The Commonwealth Government is responsible for ensuring that all Australians have access to high-quality health services and that well-educated health professionals provide these services in different locations. These locations range from public and preventative health programs to technologically sophisticated tertiary-level teaching hospitals and community-based health programs. Having an awareness of what is happening at the national level of the healthcare system will improve your health literacy competencies; it will also raise your awareness of how national policy influences what happens, for example, in service delivery at the state and organisational levels. Improving your health literacy skills will ensure that in your interactions with the patient/consumer and their families or carers you will be able to either access relevant information for them or direct them to more appropriate service providers. Familiarising yourself with Department of Health websites will alert you to what health research programs are being funded and the priority areas in health services for government.

Australia's healthcare system is a mix of public and private health service providers. Through fund allocation to the states and territories, the Commonwealth Government controls the development and management of health services through the **National Healthcare Agreement (NHA)**. The principal objective of this agreement is 'to improve the health outcomes for all Australians and the sustainability of the Australian health system' (Council of Australian Governments (CoAG), 2014). The NHA clearly articulates the scope of the agreement; its objectives and outcomes; and the joint Commonwealth, and state and territory responsibilities, as well as those specific to each state and territory. The NHA is very clear about the expected health and organisational outcomes that government funding is used for, and requires that each state and territory government make transparent the outcomes of their operational activities within their health services.

Australia's healthcare system has undergone numerous reforms over the decades, with the aims of developing efficiencies, and improving equity and access to healthcare services for all citizens. During your undergraduate program, no doubt there will have been some mention of reforms. In 2009 the National Health and Hospitals Reform Commission (NHHRC) report, *A healthier future for all Australians* was published. This document commissioned by the then federal Labor government is the blueprint for transforming Australia's fragmented healthcare system into an integrated system. The authors of the report note that Australia's healthcare system is under pressure because of changing demographic trends and associated healthcare needs, increasing concerns about the safety of healthcare services, and long waiting lists for services, reflecting access issues and ongoing equity issues. There were over one hundred recommendations in the report, including tackling access and equity issues in areas such as mental

NATIONAL HEALTHCARE AGREEMENT (NHA) – The National Healthcare Agreement (NHA) defines the goals of the health system. It specifies the roles and responsibilities of the Commonwealth and State governments in improving health outcomes for Australians and ensuring sustainability of the health system. The seven objectives of the National Healthcare Agreements are prevention; primary and community health; hospital and related care; aged care; patient experience; social inclusion and indigenous health and sustainability (CoAG, 2014).

and dental health, redesigning the healthcare system with greater emphasis on health promotion and primary health care services, and changes to the role and responsibilities of the Commonwealth and state governments in the funding and delivery of healthcare services (NHHRC, 2009).

These issues, alongside perceptions of impending health workforce shortages, particularly in medicine and nursing, are situated within concerns by government and/or policy-makers about the impact of 'population ageing' on the supply and demand for health professionals and the healthcare system (Commonwealth of Australia, 2010). Australian Government heavily influences discussion around demand for, and supply of, healthcare workers, and the nature of the services they provide. Government regulates, and are major employers of, health workers (Duckett & Willcox, 2011). Collectively, the federal, state, and territory governments provided 69.7 per cent of the 140.2 billion dollars (9.5 per cent of GDP) spent on healthcare in Australia in 2011–2012. The remainder ($42.4 billion, or 30.3 per cent of total funding) was provided by the non-government sector that comprises individuals, private health insurers, and workers' compensation (AIHW, 2013).

Critical reflection

Access the Commonwealth Government's Department of Health website at www. health.gov.au and look at the information available to you. Select one or two items that are relevant to you in your practice and discuss these in your study groups. Access the website of your state or territory's department of health and look at the programs and initiatives that are occurring or are planned to occur. Which of these programs or initiatives are going to influence your future practice in the short term? Which will influence your future practice in the long term?

Australia's Healthcare Workforce

The Australian Institute of Health and Welfare (AIHW), Australia's national agency for health and welfare statistics and information, uses two approaches to define the healthcare workforce—occupations that are health-related and industry. Health-related occupations include medical practitioners (General Practitioners (GPs) and specialists), nurses and midwives, and allied health professionals and other healthcare workers. Health services industries cover the provision of hospital services (including psychiatric hospitals); medical services; pathology and diagnostic imaging services; and allied health services. Industries outside health care, notably aged care and child care services, are excluded (AIHW 2012).

The most powerful healthcare professional group is doctors and, among them, differences exist; for example, differences between GPs and the various specialities. Doctors' interests are served by each speciality's professional college (e.g. the Royal Australasian College of Physicians (RACP) and the Royal Australasian College of Surgeons (RACS)), as well as by the Australian Medical Association (AMA), a professional association that also has an industrial function. There are also local state-based unions, such as the Salaried Medical Officers Association, the union which negotiates enterprise bargaining agreements between salaried medical officers and their employers (Willis et al. 2004). Of Australia's 91,504 doctors, the majority work as clinicians (94.5 per cent), with the largest group of these being specialists (35.0 per cent) closely followed by GPs (34.5 per cent). Over two-fifths (46.4 per cent) of doctors work in private practice, with 71.2 per cent working in group practices and 27.1 per cent in solo practices (AIHW, 2014). Doctors working in private practice are paid on a fee-for-services basis, while those working in the public sector are salaried medical officers or staff medical officers (SMOs) and private practice consultants— referred to as 'visiting medical officers' (VMOs). These doctors are paid on a sessional or contract basis (Willis et al. 2004).

Nurses are by far the largest group of healthcare professionals. The nursing workforce is discussed in some detail later in this chapter. Nurses' professional interests are met by the Australian College of Nursing and the national Australian Nursing and Midwifery Federation (ANMF) or union. The ANMF serves both nurses' professional and industrial interests.

Allied health professionals include audiologists, chiropractors, dietitians, exercise physiologists, genetic counsellors, music therapists, occupational therapists, orthotists/prosthetists, osteopaths, pharmacists, physiotherapists, podiatrists, perfusionists, psychologists, social workers, sonographers and speech pathologists (AHPA, 2014). Allied health professionals work in private practice, and in public and private hospitals and health centres. Private health insurers may reimburse the services of some allied health professionals such as chiropractors and physiotherapists. Furthermore, allied health professionals may be categorised into those that diagnose and engage in private practice, such as psychologists, and those that perform procedures directly under the control of doctors, for instance, radiologists. Allied health professionals also have their professional associations (Willis et al. 2004).

As of 1 July 2010, the Health Practitioner Regulation National Law (the National Law) is in force in each state and territory; it regulates 14 health professions through a national registration and accreditation scheme. These professions are: Aboriginal and Torres Strait Islanders health professionals, Chinese medicine, chiropractors, dental practitioners, medical practitioners, medical radiation practitioners, such as radiographers, nurses and midwives, occupational therapists, pharmacists, podiatrists and psychologists (AHPRA 2014). A defining feature of health is the highly feminised nature of the workforce, with women dominating in nursing and midwifery, and allied health (AIHW, 2012).

A recent Health Workforce Australia report (HWA 2012) identified a number of issues facing Australia's health workforce, including the mal-distribution of medical practitioners across the country, insufficient specialist training places for medical graduates, a significant nursing shortage, with areas of mental health and aged care being particularly at risk, and Australia's dependency on international doctors and nurses for its workforce. Australia's nursing workforce will be discussed in the next section.

Australia's nursing workforce

Nurses and midwives in Australia are registered as nurses, midwives or both (AIHW, 2013). The 2013, *Nursing and Midwifery Workforce report* (AIHW 2013) indicated that in 2012, there were 334,078 registered nurses and midwives in Australia with the majority employed in nursing or midwifery (93.2 per cent); a high workforce participation rate. Nursing in Australia is a female-dominated and ageing profession. In 2012, women comprised 89.8 per cent of employed nurses and midwives, with only 10.2 per cent of nurses being male (AIHW, 2013). The proportion of male registered nurses (10.4 per cent) increased between the years 2008 and 2012 (up from 9.7 per cent in 2008) over this same period of time, as did the proportion of male enrolled nurses: 8.7 per cent in 2008 to 9.2 per cent in 2012 (AIHW, 2013). Most of Australia's nurses work part-time (i.e. less than 35 hours per week). In the 2011 census, 51 per cent of female nurses and one-quarter (26 per cent) of male nurses worked part-time (ABS, 2013). The average age of the world's nursing workforce is increasing. In Australia, the average age of employed nurses is calculated as 44.6 years for registered nurses and 46.0 years for enrolled nurses. The average age of nurses increased slightly in 2008–2012 from 44.1 years in 2008 to 44.6 years, and the proportion of nurses and midwives aged 50 years or older increased from 35.1 per cent to 39.1 per cent in 2012 (AIHW, 2013). This increase in the proportion of mature nurses has implications for employers and for nurse retention. With many nurses approaching retirement age, this raises concerns that there will be not only insufficient numbers of experienced nurses taking their place but also a loss of nursing expertise (ICN, 2008), factors that will contribute to and deepen the nursing shortage.

Most nurses are clinicians providing direct care to patients, with other nurses working in administration, as educators or as researchers. In 2012, the majority of nurses and midwives employed in Australia worked as clinicians (80.1 per cent). Of these, 62.6 per cent worked in hospitals and 12.2 per cent in residential aged care facilities (AIHW, 2013). Therefore, it is highly likely that you may be working in a hospital or residential aged care facility following graduation. As an indication of the numbers of nurses working in Australia's public and private hospitals in the period 2011–2012, nurses made up 46 per cent of the full-time staff in public hospitals. Salaried medical officers comprised 13 per cent of full-time staff, and diagnostic and allied health professionals comprised 14 per cent. In the private sector, the hospital staffing mix is somewhat different, primarily because medical services are not provided by the hospital's staff. Nurses working in private hospitals also make up the largest staffing category (57 per cent) with medical officers, and diagnostic and allied health professionals comprising 7 per cent of full-time staff (AIHW, 2013).

Nurse staffing: organising work

Over the past decade, healthcare in Australia, as in many countries around the world, has seen a number of reforms in the delivery and financing of health services. These reforms have resulted in significant changes to how healthcare is delivered, with much attention drawn to the shortage of nurses worldwide (WHO, 2006; ICN, 2010, Tourangeau et al. 2010, Juraschek et al. 2012, Sherman et al. 2013).

A number of reports specific to Australia relate to nurses' working conditions, and the relation of this to nurse retention and recruitment, including recent government inquiries describing the present nursing shortage; all predicting a worsening situation (Garling, 2008; National Health Workforce Taskforce (NHWT), 2009; Productivity Commission, 2005). It is in this context of a recognised, global nursing shortage that the issue of workloads in nursing becomes a subject for considerable discussion.

Questions surrounding nurse staffing levels and skill mix (Roche et al. 2012, Aiken et al. 2013), the use of temporary or agency staff (Hurst & Smith, 2011), along with concerns with nurse numbers in relation to patient safety and risk, nurses' professional roles, and the extent to which nursing might be and/or is valued is well reported (Duffield et al. 2007, Graham & Duffield, 2010, Twigg et al. 2012). All these questions are set against a backdrop of cost pressures that will shape how you work.

Perceptions of impending health workforce shortages, and in nursing in particular, are situated within concerns by government and/or policy-makers about the impact of an ageing workforce on the supply and demand for health professionals and the healthcare system (HWA, 2012). Duckett and Willcox (2011) argue that some of the issues with determining the number of nurses needed for care delivery are related to a lack of clarification of the professional nursing role. Without this role clarification, educational institutions cannot design appropriate curricula or determine the numbers of students that need to be enrolled in nurse education programs (Duckett & Willcox 2011, p. 92).

Nursing workforce issues are longstanding. For example, in the ten years from 2004 to 2014, federal, state and territory governments commissioned numerous reports relating to nursing recruitment, retention and training (see, for example, Garling 2008; NHWT, 2009; Preston, 2006) to attempt to address nursing workforce issues. In an effort to make Australia's health workforce more responsive to the nation's health needs, the government, acting on recommendations outlined in the Productivity Commission (2005) report into the health workforce, legislated for the establishment of Health Workforce Australia, in July 2009, through the *Health Workforce Australia Act 2009* (Cth). This is a national workforce authority to support workforce planning and policy development, and manage health reform.

Other factors that impact on addressing health workforce needs and have particular relevance for registered nurses and midwives are **professional skills escalation** and expansion of the scope of practice, such as nurse practitioners and clinical nurse specialist roles.

Flexible work practices

Australia's health workforce is facing significant challenges (HWA, 2012). As noted earlier in this chapter, these challenges include not only those of an ageing population, increased demand for, and expectations with health service delivery, a changing burden of disease but also broader issues of healthcare workforce shortages, and managing those shortages such as a reliance on international healthcare professionals (HWA, 2012). Healthcare organisations manage some of these workforce challenges at the local level by engaging in business management strategies of downsizing and reengineering, and in flexibility practices. For instance, by reducing the number of registered nurses employed, through workforce substitution— **functional flexibility**. **Numerical flexibility** is attained through practices where nurses' working time is adjusted by asking or requiring part-time/full-time staff to work overtime and/or take time off due to fluctuating patient occupancy levels. Other numerical flexibility practices include limiting the duration of hours worked through increased use of agency or casual staff, asking nurses to come in to work on their days off or being 'on call'. These practices have resulted in intensification of nurses' work and workload, with increased **hospital errors** and reduced staff morale (Duffield et al. 2009, Carryer et al. 2011, Jacob et al. 2013).

PROFESSIONAL SKILLS ESCALATION – The expectations of people's performance in their jobs. Organisations are demanding greater skills, flexibility and performance of their staff during the time they are at work. This is also referred to as 'work intensification'.

FUNCTIONAL FLEXIBILITY – Role substitution such as replacing registered and/or enrolled nurses with less skilled healthcare workers, such as nurse assistants.

NUMERICAL FLEXIBILITY – Attained through practices where nurses' working time is adjusted by asking or requiring part-time/full-time staff to work overtime and/or take time off due to fluctuating patient occupancy levels.

HOSPITAL ERROR – Errors that occur in treatment of a patient during an episode of care while in hospital.

Another factor that influences workforce expectations is the notion of **work-life balance**, the idea that workforce participation must be held in balance with an individual's personal and family commitments. Workforce expectations in the healthcare sector are also related to the generational aspects of the workforce (see chapter 2).

Changes to Service Delivery

Changes to health services provision may result in significant changes to the way nurses practise, as well as changing where nurses practise. For instance, as you know from your undergraduate program, chronic disease management now occurs outside of healthcare facilities, either in the community and/or at patients' homes.

During your clinical placements, you will have noticed the different models of service delivery in the various healthcare organisations you spent time in as a student nurse. Policy directives drive changes in service delivery, changes to medical technologies (such as pharmaceuticals and diagnostic technologies) and the impact of evidence-based research are all contributors to changes in service delivery. Another important element that determines the level and type of service delivery model is the availability of appropriately skilled and qualified health professionals.

Changes in technologies will also impact on the way health services are delivered. However, while health technologies are increasing life expectancies by improving diagnostic capacities, these technologies come at a cost. Advances in health technologies will require new skills and competencies and make changes to the way health services are managed and delivered. Web-based technologies used in treating health conditions will also change the way in which health services are delivered.

eHealth

The Australian community has had access to, and demands quality healthcare services and there are expectations that this will continue. However, escalating demand for health services, coupled with a tightening/diminishing health workforce, is currently making timely access for individuals problematic.

As beginning registered nurses it is important for you to understand how the healthcare system is evolving also in light of increased consumer **health literacy**. Electronic and communication technologies (**eHealth**) and increased use of mobile device technologies (**mHealth**) to access healthcare, open up opportunities for the provision of nursing and health services in different and innovative ways: ways

WORK-LIFE BALANCE — The balance between work and personal life.

HEALTH LITERACY — The knowledge and skills required to understand and use information relating to health issues.

eHEALTH — the combined use of communication and information technology in the healthcare sector to deliver the right information to the right person at the right time in a secure electronic environment, to ensure the optimal delivery of safe, quality care to patients. eHealth is the infrastructure that supports information exchange between all healthcare professionals and patients.

mHEALTH — Healthcare services that are accessed by mobile devices such as mobile phones, smartphones, laptops and tablets to collect, retrieve and/or deliver health information.

that move care into cyberspace and patients into virtual medical (and nursing) practices (Boisvert, 2012). These ways may potentially provide cost-effective and time-saving health and nursing services. Social networks such as Facebook, patient portals, YouTube, and electronic record platforms all have the potential to alter relationships between doctors, nurses and patients wherever they may be.

Despite the reported benefits of using eHealth and its associated technologies, for example, in managing chronic conditions (Fairbrother et al. 2014, Harris et al. 2012), there remain barriers to its uptake. Barriers include a lack of awareness and confidence with using technologies by healthcare professionals and patients alike, and concerns with security and privacy (Brewster et al. 2014; Harvey & Harvey 2014).

Electronic and communication technologies are an integral part of your nursing practice now and into the future. These technologies are represented in your nursing practice standards (competencies) and, in terms of your employability, they will be found in your job description and/or contract of employment.

You may wish to consider how, as a new registered nurse, you are going to manage increased patient expectations, patient knowledge and the technologies that are making all of this possible.

Critical reflection

Australia is in the process of implementing a national shared electronic health record system and people are encouraged to register for a personally controlled electronic health record — an eHealth record. What do you think are the advantages of using such a system for nursing? There has been little uptake by Australian's of eHealth records despite incentives, particularly to GPs to do so. Why do you think this may be?

A patient asks you whether they should register for an eHealth record, as they are concerned that their records will not remain private. How will you respond?

Workforce specialisation

From your clinical placement experiences, you will have noted the diversity and specialist nature of the healthcare workforce. Even non-clinical staff are becoming increasingly specialised, moving from general administrative services to more specialist human resources services, finance services, information technology services and consumer advocate personnel. There is potential for increased workforce specialisation in the future because of the new technologies being introduced into health services delivery. These new technologies have the potential to prolong life and to halt or slow down disease processes, which in turn has the potential to change the practice of nursing.

Nursing is becoming increasingly specialised, and this is evident in the clinical specialisations that nurses now work in. The more obvious clinical specialisations for nurses include critical care nursing, emergency department nursing, renal nursing, cardiovascular nursing, aged care nursing, community nursing, and nurse practitioner in a clinical specialty. You may have already decided which nursing specialisation you wish to go into, or you may use the TPPP to help you make this decision. In making this decision, you will find out about the specific entry criteria required, what further studies you will be required to complete, and the registration and any other professional requirements you will need to meet. Because entry into these specific clinical specialisations is tightly controlled, you may find that the fluctuations in supply and demand seen elsewhere in the health workforce may not be as evident in them.

THEORY TO PRACTICE

You have a young family and are employed part-time in an acute surgical ward of a private metropolitan hospital. You chose to work at this hospital because it is 'family friendly'; you are able to organise your roster so that you are able to take or pick up your children from school. Hospital inpatient occupancy has been high over the winter months and you have been asked numerous times if you could start work earlier or leave later, and/or pick up extra shifts, including night duty. You have agreed to do so on many occasions, so as to 'help out'. Consequently, you find yourself working increasingly longer hours, occasionally ten or twelve-hour shifts, or a double shift because the ward is short staffed. Reasons put forward for the staffing shortage include sick leave and skill mix. You note that during the extra shifts you work that the ward is more often than not staffed with casuals and/or agency nurses, some of whom are rostered for short shifts—four or five hours' duration only. Although you are happy to help out and welcome the extra income, you are beginning to resent the amount of time you are spending at work.

- What flexible work practice is the organisation engaging in in this scenario and why?
- What are the implications of working these hours for the quality and safety of patient care?
- How does skill mix impact on nurse staffing?
- What are the implications of working these hours for your work-life balance?

Australia's healthcare workforce is multidisciplinary and comprises medicine, nursing and allied health staff, supported by management, administration and information technology personnel. It is defined not only by the different professional disciplines, but also by how work is structured at the broader level of the healthcare system and within the healthcare organisations in which nurses' work.

Critical reflection

- Having read through this chapter, what do you think are the three most significant issues facing Australia's healthcare system?
- What are the implications of these issues for nursing?
- As beginning registered nurse, how do you think that these issues will impact on how you do your job/work?

SUMMARY

This chapter discusses how Australia's healthcare system is funded and managed at the national, state and territory levels. While this may seem like abstract or 'dry' information, you should at least have an awareness of how the healthcare system is organised and be familiar with the national and state and territory departments that manage it. You should keep up to date, through the media, with the federal government's proposed changes to the healthcare system.

This chapter also looks at health workforce issues, especially the nurse shortage. Being aware of nurse workforce issues will help you to understand the issues you will face in your own workplace and why staffing shifts in your workplace is a complex task. This chapter has been written to contextualise the healthcare workplace for you and to help you understand that the issues you are facing are also being faced by other healthcare professionals, as well as nurses in other parts of the country.

Discussion questions

1. What are the key issues facing Australia's healthcare system?
2. How important is it for you to know about how the healthcare system operates?
3. In a group, discuss the healthcare organisations as a system.
4. What are the immediate connections you can see within your organisation?

5. In a group, reflect on the technologies you were introduced to as a student nurse in the clinical skills laboratories and clinical placement. What were your immediate reactions when you were asked to work with the piece of equipment or technology? Where was your attention focused: the patient or the technology?

Further Reading

Currie, EJ, & Carr-Hill, RA 2013, 'What is a nurse? Is there an international consensus?', *International Nursing Review*, vol. 60, no. 1, pp. 67–74, doi:10.1111/j.1466-7657.2012 .00997.x.

Melon, KA, White D, & Rankin, J 2013, 'Beat the clock! Wait times and the production of 'quality' in emergency departments', *Nursing Philosophy*, vol. 14, no. 3 pp. 223–7, doi:10 .1111/nup.12022.

Newman, S & Lawler, J 2009, 'Managing healthcare under new public management: a Sisyphean challenge for nursing', *Journal of Sociology*, vol. 45, no. 4, pp. 419–32, doi:10 .1177/1440783309346477.

West, S, Mapedzahama, V, Ahern, M, & Rudge, T 2013, 'Rethinking shift work: midlife nurses making it work!', *Nursing Inquiry*, vol. 19, no. 2, pp. 177–87, doi:10.1111/j .1440-1800.2011.00552.x.

Urban, A 2014, 'Taken for granted: normalizing nurses' work in hospitals', *Nursing Inquiry* vol. 21, no.1, pp. 69–78, doi:10.1111/nin.12033.

Useful websites

Australian Government Department of Health for all information about the role of the Department, including departmental structures, annual reports, budgets, legislation and policy pertaining to the Australian healthcare system: http://www.health.gov.au.

Australian Health Practitioner Regulation Agency (AHPRA) the organisation responsible for the implementation of the National Registration and Accreditation Scheme across Australia. It is the single regulatory authority for 14 health professions: http://www. ahpra.gov.au/.

Health Workforce Australia (HWA) is a Commonwealth statutory authority. It was established by the Council of Australian Governments (CoAG) to address health workforce issues and reforms to meets the healthcare needs of Australians: https://www. hwa.gov.au/.

International Council of Nurses (ICN) represents the interests of nursing internationally in areas such as professional practice, nurse regulation and nursing, health and social policy: http://www.icn.ch.

Nursing and Midwifery Board of Australia is the national nursing and midwifery regulatory authority under the National Registration and Accreditation Scheme: http:// www.nursingmidwiferyboard.gov.au.

MARIA FEDORUK AND LUISA TOFFOLI

References

Aiken, LH, Slone, DM, Bruyneel, L, Van den Heede, K & Sermeus, W for the RN4CAST Consortium (2013) 'Nurses' reports of working conditions and hospital quality of care in 12 countries in Europe', *International Journal of Nursing Studies*, vol. 50, no. 2, pp. 143–53.

Allied Health Professions Australia (AHPA) 'About us', viewed 28 March 2014 http://www .ahpa.com.au/Home/aboutAHPA.aspx.

Australian Bureau of Statistics (ABS), 2013. 4102.0 – *Australian Social Trends*, April 2013, viewed 28 March 2014 http://www.abs.gov.au/AUSSTATS/abs@.nsf/ Lookup/4102.0Main+Features20April+2013#p3.

Australian Institute of Health & Welfare 2012, *Australia's health 2012*. Australia's health no. 13. Cat. no. AUS 156. Canberra.

Australian Institute of Health and Welfare 2013, *Health expenditure Australia 2011–12*, Health and welfare expenditure series no. 50. Cat. no. HWE 59. Canberra.

Australian Institute of Health and Welfare 2013, *Nursing and midwifery workforce 2012*, National health workforce series no. 6. Cat. no. HWL 52. Canberra.

Australian Institute of Health and Welfare 2014, *Medical Workforce 2012*, National health workforce series no. 8. Cat. no. HWL 54. Canberra.

Boisvert, S 2012, 'Getting to zero: technology. An enterprise look at mHealth', *Journal of Healthcare Risk Management*, vol.32, no.2, pp. 44–52, DOI: 10.1002/jhrm.

Brewster, L, Mountain, G, Wessels, B, Kelly, C & Hawley, M 2014, 'Factors affecting front line staff acceptance of telehealth technologies: a mixed-method systematic review', *Journal of Advanced Nursing*, vol. 70, no.1, pp. 21–33.

Buerhaus, PI, Auerbach, DI, Staiger, DO & Muench, U 2013, 'Projections of the long-term growth of the registered nurse workforce: a regional analysis',*Nursing Economics*, vol. 31, no. 1, pp. 13–17.

Carryer, JB, Diers, AD, McCloskey, B & Wilson, D 2011, 'Effects of health policy reforms on nursing resources and patient outcomes in New Zealand', *Policy, Politics and Nursing Practice*, vol. 11, no. 4, pp. 275–85.

Commonwealth of Australia 2010, *Intergenerational report. Australia to 2050: future challenges*, Attorney-General's Department, Canberra, viewed 29 March 2014 http:// www.treasury.gov.au.

Commonwealth of Australia 2012, *Health Workforce Australia Act 2009*, viewed 27 March 2014 http://www.comlaw.gov.au/Details/C2012C00032.

Council of Australian Governments (CoAG) 2014, *National healthcare agreement 2012 Australian Government*, Canberra, viewed 27 March 2014 http://www. federalfinancialrelations.gov.au/content/npa/healthcare/national-agreement.pdf.

Department of Education, Science and Training 2002, *National review of nursing education*, Nursing Education Review Secretariat, Canberra, DEST No. 6880 HERC02A.

Duckett, S & Willcox, S 2011, *The Australian health care system*, 4th edn, Oxford University Press, Melbourne.

Duffield, C, Diers, D, Aisbett, C & Roche, M 2009, 'Churn: patient turnover and casemix', *Nursing Economic$*, 27(3), 185–91.

Duffield, L, Roche, M, O'Brien-Pallas, L, Diers, D, Aisbett, C, Aisbett, K, King, M & Hall, J 2007, *Gluing it together: nurses, their work environment and patient safety*, report prepared for NSW Health: University of Technology Sydney.

Fairbrother, P, Ure, J, Hanley, J, McCloughan, L, Denvir, M, Sheikh, A, McKinstry, B & the Telescot programme team 2014, 'Telemonitoring for chronic heart failure: the views of patients and healthcare professionals—a qualitative study', *Journal of Clinical Nursing*, vol. 23, no. 1–2, pp. 132–44, doi: 10.1111/jocn.12137.

Garling, P 2008, *Final report of the special commission of inquiry: acute care in NSW public hospitals, 2008 Volume 1*, State of NSW through the Special Commission of Inquiry: Acute Care Services in New South Wales Public Hospitals viewed 27 March 2014 http://www.dpc.nsw.gov.au/__data/assets/pdf_file/0005/34187/Volume_1_-_Special_Commission_Of_Inquiry_Into_Acute_Care_Services_In_New_South_Wales_Public_Hospitals.pdf.

Graham, EM & Duffield, C 2010, 'An ageing nursing workforce', *Australian Health Review*, vol. 34, no. 1, pp. 44–8.

Harris, MA, Hood, KK, & Mulvaney, SS 2012, 'Pumpers, skypers, surfers and texters: technology to improve the management of diabetes in teenagers', *Diabetes, Obesity and Metabolism*, vol. 14, no. 11, pp. 967–72, doi: 10.1111/j.1463-1326.2012.01599.x.

Harvey, MJ & Harvey, MG 2014, 'Privacy and security issues for mobile health platforms', *Journal of the Association for Information Science and Technology*, doi: 10.1002/asi.23066.

Health Workforce Australia 2012, *Health Workforce 2025— Doctors, Nurses and Midwives— Volume 1*, Health Workforce Australia, Adelaide viewed 27 March 2014 http://www.hwa.gov.au/sites/uploads/FinalReport_Volume1_FINAL-20120424.pdf

Hurst, K & Smith, A 2011, 'Temporary nursing staff— cost and quality issues', *Journal of Advanced Nursing*, vol. 67, no. 2, pp. 287–96 doi: 10.1111/j.1365-2648.2010.05471.x.

International Council of Nurses 2006, *The global nursing shortage: priority areas for intervention*, The Council, Geneva.

International Council of Nurses 2008, *An ageing nursing workforce*, The Council, Geneva viewed 29 March 2014 http://www.icn.ch/images/stories/documents/publications/fact_sheets/2a_FS-Ageing_Workforce.pdf.

Jacob, ER, McKenna, L & D'Amore, A 2013, 'The changing skill mix in nursing: consideration for and against different levels of nurse', *Journal of Nursing Management*, doi:10.1111/jonm.12162.

Juraschek, S, Zhang, X, Ranganathan, V & Lin, VW 2012, 'United States registered nurse workforce report card and shortage forecast', *American Journal of Medical Quality*, vol. 27 no. 3, pp. 241–9, doi: 10.1177/1062860611416634.

National Health and Hospitals Reform Commission 2009, *A healthier future for all Australians*, Final Report June 2009, Commonwealth of Australia, Canberra, viewed 27 March 2014, http://www.health.gov.au/internet/nhhrc/publishing.nsf/content/1AFDEAF1FB76A1D8CA257600000B5BE2/$File/Final_Report_of_the%20nhhrc_June_2009.pdf.

National Health Workforce Taskforce (NHWT) 2009, *Health Workforce in Australia and Factors for Current Shortages*, KPMG, Melbourne, viewed 27 March 2014 http://www.ahwo.gov.au/documents/NHWT/The%20health%20workforce%20in%20Australia%20and%20factors%20influencing%20current%20shortages.pdf.

Preston, B 2006, *Nurse Workforce Futures: development and application of a model of demand and supply of graduates of Australian and New Zealand pre-registration nursing and midwifery courses to 2010*. Council of Deans of Nursing and Midwifery (Australia & New Zealand, Melbourne viewed 27 March 2014 http://www.cdnm.edu.au/wp-content/uploads/2011/09/Nurseworkforcefutures.pdf.

Productivity Commission 2005, *Australia's health workforce*, Research Report, Canberra, viewed 27 March 2014 http://www.pc.gov.au/__data/assets/pdf_file/0003/9480/healthworkforce.pdf

Roche, M, Duffield, C, Aisbett, C, Diers, D & Stasa, H 2012, 'Nursing work directions in Australia: does evidence drive the policy?' *Collegian*, vol. 19, no. 4, pp. 231–8

Sherman, RO, Chiang-Hanisko, L & Koszalinski, R 2013, 'The ageing nursing workforce: a global challenge' *Journal of Nursing Management*, vol. 21, no.7, pp. 899–902, doi: 10.1111/jonm.12188.

Tourangeau, AE, Cummings, G, Cranley, LA, Ferron, EM & Harvey, S 2010, 'Determinants of hospital nurse intention to remain employed: broadening our understanding', *Journal of Advanced Nursing*, vol. 66, no. 1, pp. 22–32, doi:10.1111/j.1365-2648.2009.05190.x.

Twigg, D, Duffield, C, Bremner, A, Rapley, P & Finn, J 2012, 'Impact of skill mix variations on patient outcomes following implementation of nursing hours per patient day staffing: a retrospective study,' *Journal of Advanced Nursing*, vol. 68, no. 12, pp. 2710–18, doi:10.1111/j.1365-2648.2012.05971.

Willis, E, Young, S & Stanton, P 2005, 'Health sector and industrial reform in Australia', in P Stanton, E Willis, & S Young (Eds), *Workplace reform in the healthcare industry; the Australian experience*, pp. 13–29, Palgrave MacMillan, London, England.

World Health Organization (WHO) 2006, *Working together for health*, World Health Report. viewed 31 March 2014 http://www.who.int/whr/2006/en

Leadership in Nursing and Health Care

8

MARIA FEDORUK

LEARNING OBJECTIVES

After reading this chapter, you will be able to:

- define leadership
- apply leadership principles to your own practice
- explain why nurses need to be leaders
- apply the principles of emotional intelligence and social intelligence to yourself.

KEY TERMS

Clinical leadership
Emotional intelligence
Followership
Leadership
Transformational leadership

Introduction

This chapter provides you with an overview of **leadership** and its application to nurses and to nursing practice. McKee, Kemp and Spence (2013, p. 19) note that leadership can be learned, and all people can learn how to lead by incorporating their values, beliefs, knowledge and experiences into their daily life and work. Nurses need to develop leadership competencies because nurses manage the patient care environment, and exercise leadership 'during their interactions with patients, their families and with professional colleagues' (Curtis et al. 2011, p. 344). Leadership has been described as an 'art and science' by Barr and Dowding (2013, p. 4). Leadership is an art because there are many aspects of leadership that cannot be learned, a fact contradicted by McKee, Kemp and Spence (2013). Leadership is a science, because a growing body of knowledge is reporting on the many and varied processes that contribute to leadership. One of the barriers to defining leadership is the 'belief that leadership is related to seniority' (Barr & Dowding 2013, p. 4). This belief is still apparent in many healthcare organisations, especially in nursing organisations.

LEADERSHIP — Seeing what is in the present, seeing what needs to be done and closing the gap (adapted from GG Cummings).

TRANSFOR-
MATIONAL
LEADERSHIP – A
participative style
of leadership that
motivates others to
achieve goals beyond
expectations.

Leadership as a concept and a construct has been written about and discussed for many years, and the leadership theories that have been developed over the past century have ranged from the 'command and control' style (military antecedents) to the more contemporary behavioural styles of leadership such as **transformational leadership**. Transformational leadership is a more participative style of leadership and the transformational leader 'values results and outcomes', values, interprofessional and intraprofessional relationships with colleagues and inspires followers to achieve goals beyond expectations by focusing on achievements and being empowered to do so (Dwyer & Hopwood 2013, p. 237). At the core of transformational leadership is the notion of emotional intelligence.

Critical reflection

Reflect on a time in your life when you assumed a leadership role. This could be while you were still at school or part of a sports team. What factors indicated to you that you were in a leadership role?

Leadership and Emotional Intelligence

EMOTIONAL
INTELLIGENCE –
Having self-
awareness, social
awareness, able to
manage relationships
and able to
manage self.

Emotional intelligence is a multifaceted phenomenon first identified in the early 1990s by Mayer and Salovey (Cummings et al. 2010). Their seminal research defined emotional intelligence (EI) as four 'specific, interrelated abilities to deal with their own and others' emotions' (Walter, Humphrey & Cole 2012, p. 213). Because nurses are frontline workers in the healthcare system, managing emotions is integral to nursing work. Nurses work every day in emotionally charged environments, delivering care to patients whose emotions can be extremely changeable during an episode of care. The dynamic nature of healthcare environments (think about a day in a hospital ward and the chaos that nurses work with) emphasises the emotional nature of nursing work from both the nurse and patient perspective. The highs and lows caused by emotion can affect your decision-making and, hence, patient outcomes. Emotions can negatively affect the quality of communication between health professionals and can lead to misunderstanding and error.

Emotional intelligence was made popular in 1995 by Daniel Goleman, a journalist who defined it as having four pillars:

1. self-awareness
2. self-regulation
3. empathy
4. social skills (Goleman 1995).

McKee, Kemp and Spence (2013, p. 23) have broadened Goleman's work:

- emotional awareness
- social awareness
- relationship management
- self-management.

As you can see from this second explanation, 'social and emotional intelligence competencies enable people to manage their own and others' emotions in social interactions and, if you think about it, nursing practice is also a social interaction. Your professional interactions with colleagues also have elements of social interactions. Effective leadership therefore depends on developing and mastering social and emotional intelligence competencies (McKee et al. 2013, p. 20).

Critical reflection

Think about a situation (it could be on clinical placement) where you used your social and emotional intelligence competencies to manage a difficult situation. What were the outcomes, if any?

Leadership and Nurses

Health Workforce Australia (HWA) has produced a number of publications and media presentations on leadership especially for nurses in Australia, and the following link will take you to a video presentation on models of leadership presented by senior health managers and a professor of nursing: https://www.hwa.gov.au/search/node/leadership.

However, what is important to remember is that leaders and, therefore, leadership cannot exist without followers (Barr & Dowding 2013). As a student nurse you will have taken on the **followership** role as you developed your knowledge and competencies. But once you have entered the healthcare workplace, the expectations placed on you will change and you will be expected to demonstrate leadership and management competencies. Management competencies will centre around organising patient activities such as admission, discharge and preparation for procedures. The leadership dimensions of your role will focus on developing a team culture, as a team leader and as a team member. You will demonstrate leadership competencies in your interactions with diverse groups of people and in your commitment to providing safe, quality care to patients using the national approach (National Safety and Quality Health Service Standards—NSQHSS) to inform your practice. It is in the area of safety and quality that nurses can and

FOLLOWERSHIP – the process of following leaders. Leadership and followership are interdependent.

do take a strong leadership role, with nurses assuming a lead role in developing and managing safety and quality programs in health, aged care and community organisations.

Leadership in nursing and for nurses is particularly important during times of reform in health. Reforms create uncertainty around job security, impact on nurse workloads through substitution of registered nurses with less skilled workers, even though research evidence clearly identifies that registered nurses are necessary to ensure patient safety and care quality during episodes of care (Norrish & Rundall 2001; Cummings et al. 2010; Squires et al. 2010). Nurses are central to the effective management of healthcare organisations, especially in the safe, competent provision of direct care to patients. As student nurses you should take every opportunity to develop your leadership competencies, as you move through your undergraduate program and then into the registered nurse role. An effect of hospital restructuring is a de-emphasising of the nurse–patient relationship, which has always been the cornerstone of nursing practice. Following a hospital restructuring, registered nurses can find themselves engaged in indirect care activities such as data collection, care planning and coordination, which is done away from the bedside. This can result in the phenomenon of missed episodes of care now being reported in the nursing literature as well as an increase in hospital error rates (Ball et al. 2014).

THEORY TO PRACTICE

As a third-year student nurse out on your final clinical placement, you find that other students on placement in the same healthcare organisation but in different clinical units often come to see you during your break times to ask you questions about clinical issues they are encountering in their placements. You are more than happy to help these students with their queries and point them in the direction of the most recent evidence relating to their particular questions and queries. There are times when registered nurses come and ask you about certain clinical issues. One day, when you are responding to a clinical issue from another nursing student, the team leader overhears your conversation and once your colleague has left, calls you into the office and tells you that you are working outside your scope of practice and that she will report you to the university facilitator. You do not begin to react negatively to the team leader's words but somehow manage to not react, nor do you try to explain your side of events but just acknowledge the team leader's comments. At the time you are upset but once you reflect on the situation you begin to analyse the event in leadership terms.

Discussion Questions

1. Did the team leader act as a leader?
2. Was there any indication the team leader was showing any emotional or social intelligence competencies?
3. In your interactions with your colleagues, did you act as a leader?
4. Will you stop responding to your colleagues' queries in the future?

However, the team leader does report the incident to your clinical facilitator and presents a slightly different version of events. The clinical facilitator then asks to speak with you privately about the incident. You are nervous about the upcoming discussion because the worst-case scenario could be removal from placement with a negative evaluation from the healthcare unit, which could affect your future employment opportunities for a TPPP. An even worse outcome for you would be to have to repeat the placement the following year.

Discussion Questions

1. How are you going to conduct yourself in the interview?
2. What competencies are you going to draw upon?
3. How are you going to defend your position?

Clinical Leadership

Clinical leadership focuses on developing initiatives with teams of clinicians to improve services to patients (Fealy et al. 2011). Clinical leaders in nursing focus on improving nursing services to patients to ensure positive health outcomes. Stoddart et al. (2014) note that clinical leadership initiatives in Scotland are policy-driven to improve the safety and quality of patient-centred care. In Garrubba et al. (2011) the literature review on clinical leadership found no specific or standard definition of leadership but rather themes that included the ability to influence peers to enable clinical performance, to support and motivate peers to achieve strategic organisational goals and objectives, to challenge existing service delivery processes and work continually to improve the safety and quality dimensions of patient and nursing care. It takes courage and knowledge to challenge historical and traditional ways of nursing practice, especially as a student or new graduate nurse. Leadership is not only about function but also about attributes that are 'present at an organisational and individual level', where clinical leaders look to continually improve current practice and to influence others to accomplish this. Clinical leadership is not specific to any one particular clinical discipline but

CLINICAL LEADERSHIP – Enables peers to act and enable clinical performance ... to improve clinical practice and for nurses it is about improving nursing practice.

MARIA FEDORUK

includes medicine, allied health and nursing. Figure 8.1 shows an overview of the NHS (UK) Leadership framework.

This framework has been based on research and may be applied to all healthcare staff at any stage of their career (NHS Leadership Framework http://www.leadershipacademy.nhs.uk/discover/leadership-framework/).

The leadership framework is not restricted to particular management or clinical roles but is more effective when all staff share the responsibility for delivering safe, quality healthcare. So, even student nurses and new graduate nurses have a role in this shared distributive form of leadership.

FIGURE 8.1 LEADERSHIP FRAMEWORK NHS

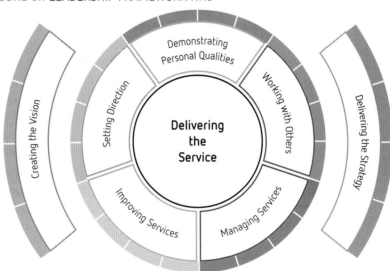

Leadership Framework overview diagram

Source: NHS Leadership Framework accessed 13 April 2014: http://www.leadershipacademy.nhs.uk/discover/leadership-framework/.

Figure 8.2 shows the Australian Leadership Framework developed by Health Workforce Australia (HWA) as a national approach to developing leadership competencies in the healthcare workforce, aligning with the national approach to safety and quality. This is a transformational leadership framework incorporating, as you can see, the EI competencies. How different is this from the NHS leadership framework (figure 8.1)? Do you think that both frameworks present healthcare leadership attributes in similar ways?

FIGURE 8.2 HWA—NATIONAL APPROACH TO LEADERSHIP IN THE HEALTHCARE SECTOR

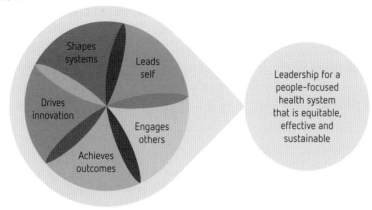

Source: Health Workforce Australia 2013. https://www.hwa.gov.au/sites/uploads/Health-LEADS-Australia-A4-FINAL.pdf

Critical reflection

In the Theory to Practice section earlier, can you see a demonstration of the elements of clinical leadership? Using the leadership frameworks in figures 8.1 and 8.2, see if you can begin to develop your own clinical leadership qualities or attributes. Where would you begin? Have you considered yourself as a clinical leader? Which framework do you find easier to work with?

Leadership for the Future

Avolio et al. (2009) reviewed the leadership literature with the aim of developing a future focus on leadership. It is important to spend some time looking to the future in relation to leadership, because while contemporary leadership is not position- or person-centred, it is context dependent. As student nurses you will be aware that the healthcare environments and contexts are dynamic and continually changing, meaning that nurse leaders have to be flexible when acting in leadership roles.

Contemporary styles of leadership include authentic leadership, shared or distributive leadership evident in the NHS leadership framework and new-genre leadership. Authentic leadership describes ethical and transparent behaviour that is inclusive of others' input into decision-making.

New-genre leadership emphasises charismatic leader behaviour, visionary ideological and moral values, as well as transformational leadership behaviours. Shared leadership is apparent where team members collectively act as leaders. It is important to note that all contemporary leadership theories take their cues from studies of emotional intelligence.

Future leadership theories will need to take into account the emerging e- and mHealth technologies now changing the context and environments of healthcare delivery. It is interesting to think how, as future nurses, you will take on the challenges posed by eHealth, which is becoming a reality. How will you manage and lead in virtual health environments, where your interactions will be mediated by technology?

SUMMARY

This chapter has provided you with an overview of leadership in nursing and in healthcare. Significantly you should now know that leadership is not vested in positions nor in seniority nor is it age related. Research studies have shown that the concept and construct of leadership is complex and widely reported in the literature, both academic and popular. Research studies from nursing and non-nursing disciplines have moved from studying leadership as a command and control construct to one of participation and inclusion.

Currently, in the healthcare and nursing literature, clinical leadership is being discussed, providing nurses, even student nurses, with opportunities to develop leadership competencies in the clinical context. In Australia, there is the Clinical Leadership Program, based on the leadership research work done in the United Kingdom. Health Workforce Australia has developed a national framework for transformational leadership development that can be used by all health professionals, including student nurses, to develop their leadership competencies.

The nursing literature (research) is showing that there are direct links between leadership in nursing and patient safety and quality outcomes. Positive nursing leadership also influences nurse retention and workforce management.

Contemporary leadership theories focus on individuals, using the attributes of EI. Challenges facing future nurse leaders include those posed by eHealth, closely followed by mHealth, where m stands for mobile. The concept of e-leadership, where groups are geographically separated and interactions are mediated by technology, will be challenging for future nurse leaders and you should reflect on them.

Discussion questions

1. What do you understand leadership to be?
2. What leadership styles have you been exposed to? How did you react or respond to these?

3. What leadership attributes do you possess? What attributes do you need to further develop your leadership skills?

4. Is it necessary for nurses to take on leadership roles in the healthcare system?

5. What do think of being a leader in a virtual environment? What competencies will you need to develop for that environment?

Further Reading

Germain, PB & Cummings, GG 2010, 'The influence of nursing leadership on nurse performance: a systematic literature review', *Journal of Nursing Management*, vol. 18, pp. 425–39.

Smith, KB, Profetto-MCGrath, J & Cummings, GG 2009, 'Emotional intelligence and nursing: an integrative review', *International Journal of Nursing Studies* vol. 46, pp. 1624–36.

Stanley, D 2011, *Clinical leadership*, Palgrave MacMillan, South Yarra, Melbourne.

Walker, RJ, Cooke, M., Henderson, A & Creedy, DK 2011, 'Characteristics of leadership that influence clinical learning: a narrative review', *Nurse Education Today*, vol. 31, pp. 743–56.

Useful websites

Clinical Excellence Commission (NSW) Clinical leadership program http://www.cec. health.nsw.gov.au/programs/clinical-leadership.

Clinical Leadership Program Australia http://www.nursingsa.com/prof_leadership.php.

Health Workforce Australia (HWA) (2013). Leadership for sustainable change. https://www.hwa.gov.au/our-work/boost-productivity/leadership-sustainable-change.

Health Workforce Australia (HWA) https://www.hwa.gov.au/search/node/leadership.

Health Workforce Australia: https://www.hwa.gov.au/resources/publications/ leadership-sustainability-health-system/leadership-sustainability-health-system-part-1. This provides a national approach (Australia) to leadership in healthcare.

Rob Goffee, Emeritus Professor of Organisational Behaviour, London Business School: https://www.hwa.gov.au/search/node/leadership.

Gareth Jones, Fellow of the Centre for Management Development, London Business School Authentic leadership and authentic organisations https://www.hwa.gov.au/news-events/ authentic-leadership-and-authentic-organisations.

The Jönköping experience—lessons learned on collaboration and leadership: https:// www.hwa.gov.au/news-events/plenary-2-j%C3%B6nk%C3%B6ping-experience-%E2%80%93-lessons-learned-collaboration-and-leadership. These links take you to videos where experienced leaders in healthcare discuss leadership in the context of contemporary healthcare organisations.

References

Avolio, BJ, Walumba, FO, &Weber, TJ 2009, 'Leadership: current theories, research, and future directions', *Annu. Rev. Pschol.*, vol. 60, pp. 421–49.

Ball, J, Murrells, T, Raffery, AM, Morrow, E & Griffiths, P 2014, ' "Care left undone" during nursing shifts: associations with workload and perceived quality of care', *BMJ Qual Saf*, vol. 23, pp. 116–25.

Barr, J & Dowding, L 2013, *Leadership in healthcare*, 2nd edn, Sage publications, London.

Cummings GG 2013, 'Nursing leadership and patient outcomes', *Journal of Nursing Management.* 21, pp. 707–8.

Cummings, GG, MacGregor, T, Davey, M, Lee How, Wong C, Lo E, Muise, M & Stafford, E 2010, 'Leadership styles and outcome patterns for the nursing workforce and work environment: a systematic review', *International Journal of Nursing Studies* 47, pp. 363–85.

Dwyer, J & Hopwood, N 2013, *Management. Strategies and skills*, 2nd edn, McGraw Hill Education (Australia) Pty Ltd.

Fealy, GM, McNamara, MS, Casey, M et al. 2011, 'Barriers to clinical leadership development: findings from a national survey', *Journal of Clinical Nursing*, 20, pp. 2023–32.

Fealy, GM, McNamara, MS, Casey, M et al. 2013, 'Service impact of a national leadership development programme: findings from a qualitative study', *Journal of Nursing Management*, pp. 1–9.

Garrubba, GM, Harris, C, Melder, A 2011, *Clinical leadership. A literature review to investigate concepts, roles and relationships related to clinical leadership*, Centre for Clinical Effectiveness, Southern Health, Melbourne Australia.

Health Workforce Australia 2013, *The national leadership framework*, https://www.hwa.gov.au/sites/uploads/Health-LEADS-Australia-A4-FINAL.pdf.

McKee, A, Kemp, T, Spence, G 2013, *Management. A focus on leaders*, Pearson Australia.

Norrish, BR & Rundall, TG 2001, 'Hospital restructuring and the work of registered nurses', *The Milbank Quarterly*, vol. 79, no. 1, pp. 55–79.

Squires, M, Tourangeau A, Laschinger, HKS & Doran D 2010, 'The link between leadership and safety outcomes in hospitals', *Journal of Nursing Management*, vol. 18, pp. 914–25.

Stoddart, K, Bugge, C, Shepherd A & Farquharson, B 2014, 'The new clinical leadership role of senior charge nurses: a mixed methods study of their views and experience', *Journal of Nursing Management*, vol. 22, pp. 49–59.

Walter, F, Humphrey, RH, Cole, MS 2012, 'Unleashing leadership potential', *Organizational Dynamics*, vol. 41, issue 3, pp. 212–19.

Wong, CA, Cummings GG & Ducharme, L 2013, 'The relationship between nursing leadership and patient outcomes: a systematic review update', *Journal of Nursing Management*, vol. 21, pp. 709–24.

Essential Competencies for the Registered Nurse

9

MARIA FEDORUK

After reading this chapter, you will be able to:

- differentiate between skills and competencies in nursing
- set priorities for your own competency development
- differentiate between management and leadership.

Communication
Competencies
Conflict management
Critical thinking
Information management
Information systems
Interprofessional conflict
Intraprofessional conflict
Management
Skills

Essential Competencies

This chapter uses the Nursing and Midwifery Board of Australia's updated and rebranded (NMBA) (2013) *National competency standards for the registered nurse* as a framework.

Chapter 12 discusses in more detail the relevance and significance of these standards to contemporary nursing practice in Australia from a legislative perspective. During your student nurse program you will have been introduced to the NMBA competency standards and their application to the practical aspects of nursing practice. This chapter discusses in broad terms what registered nurses do, while chapter 10 discusses nurses role in knowledge translation in more detail. As you may be realising by now, becoming a safe, competent registered nurse is a lifelong learning pursuit and will continue throughout your nursing career. Safe, competent registered nurses are continually learning as their environments change, the technology they use changes, their patient populations change, patient expectations change, and service delivery models change.

Skills and Competencies

SKILLS — Tasks are done well through repetition.

COMPETENCIES — Capabilities or abilities that include both intent and action that link directly to how well a person performs completing tasks.

The terms **skills** and **competencies** are often used interchangeably, but a skill is having the ability to do something well—the 'knowing how'—whereas a 'competency' is knowing how *and* knowing *why* you do something. So, a competent registered nurse not only knows how to carry out a procedure but also why the procedure is necessary. In hospital-trained nursing programs, nurses focused on task completion but did not necessarily know or understand the rationales for procedures and how these would affect patient health outcomes. There was no critical thinking attached to the completion of tasks. In contrast, in tertiary nursing studies you are not only shown how to do procedures but are also taught to understand why you are doing them. Understanding why you are doing something helps you to explain procedures to your patients and the rationale behind them. Remember that your patients have the ability to check the information you give them with other health professionals, as well as using the internet to research information. So, as a professional nurse, you must give them the correct information in a timely manner. The NMBA (2013) National Competency Standards are the core competency standards, together with the registration standards by which you will be assessed to:

- become registered
- retain your registration so that you can continue to practise as a registered nurse in Australia.

Your university will have used these standards to develop the nursing curriculum (NMBA 2013).

So you have entered the healthcare workforce at the novice level of practitioner and your aim is to become an expert in your chosen area of nursing practice. How will you become an expert in your chosen clinical area of practice? What skills and competencies will you need to continue to develop further? This is where the SMARTTA framework may help you clarify your thinking (Dwyer & Hopwood 2013, p. 261). You were introduced to the SMARTTA framework in chapter 1.

Critical reflection

SMARTTA framework
Use the SMARTTA framework to develop some learning objectives that will help you transition into the registered nurse role.

A   What will your **specific** objectives look like? A good starting point is actually being very sure of what it is you want to achieve—the end-goal—and then working backwards to develop your plan.

B   What will you use to **measure** the achievement of these objectives? What sort of criteria will you use? You could refer to the criteria of the ANMAC national competencies, or your clinical unit will have clinical indicators that you can use.

C   How **achievable** are these objectives? Do not set yourself unachievable objectives. It is always better to set objectives that are achievable (the 'baby steps' approach), otherwise you set yourself up for disappointment.

D   **How will** the objectives be **relevant** to the clinical specialty?

E   Remember **timeliness**—always set yourself timelines. This will help you maintain focus on achieving the objective, especially if one of your strategies is the completion of a professional development activity in your graduate year.

F   You also need to be able to **track** your progress, evaluating each objective as you achieve it.

G   There needs to be **agreement** with all parties involved in helping you achieve your objectives.

The following section deals with the essential skills and competencies you will need as a registered nurse to ensure your continuing registration with the Australian Health Practitioner Regulation Agency (AHPRA).

Beginning Registered Nurse Competencies

During your student nurse program, emphasis will have been placed on competency development. It is important than you continue to develop these competencies as you progress through your registered nurse career. Prospective employers expect you to provide evidence that you are a safe and competent registered nurse.

All new registered nurses must be able to demonstrate the following competencies:

- numeracy competencies
- literacy competencies
- information technology competencies
- biomedical technology competencies
- conflict management competencies
- management competencies
- leadership competencies
- interpersonal competencies.

Numeracy competencies

The most obvious nursing function for which nurses and midwives must have good numeracy skills is drug calculations and medication administration. The most common critical incidents in Australian healthcare organisations are drug errors, and nurses are predominantly responsible and accountable for giving out medications to patients. There was a reason drug calculation tests featured prominently in your undergraduate program: to make you a safe, competent registered nurse when administering medications to patients. It is a fact of nursing life—nurses are expected to give the right drug, in the right dose, to the right patient at the right time. The nursing literature indicates that medication errors by nurses are a universal phenomenon (Jordan 2011, Sherwood 2012). The outcomes of medication errors can be clinically irreversible, and costly in terms of compensation and reputation for the healthcare organisation, and can result in deregistration for the nurse. So, even though you are now a registered nurse, it is in your best interests to continue practising drug calculations. At 3 am in the morning during an emergency situation no one is going to give you a pen and paper or calculator to work out drug dosages. This is called 'the 3am rule'.

While accuracy in drug administration is important in adult nursing, it is particularly important in neonatal and paediatrics nursing, where drug dosages are calculated per gram or kilogram of the infant's body weight.

Another area of medication management where you will need good numeracy skills is managing intravenous therapies containing medications that need to be titrated against biochemical results or against body weight, or even against changes in clinical symptoms. In these instances, you will also be monitoring insertion sites for the intravenous therapies for infections, inflammation dislodgement or clotting—all of which can affect the accuracy of the drug administration to a particular patient.

Drug administration is not the only area of nursing and clinical practice where numeracy skills are necessary. Numeracy skills are necessary when:

- working out blood results and noting any abnormality that has to be reported to medical staff because changes to treatment are indicated (other examples include when looking after respiratory-compromised patients where correct oxygen concentrations are essential, in cardiac patients where abnormal levels of potassium need treating)
- calculating body mass index
- counting patient's money on admission, especially where the patient's mental state is compromised
- calculating percentage of burns suffered by patients
- calculating the number of staff needed for safe practice on a shift
- calculating patient dependency levels
- reading and interpreting research results.

As a registered nurse, if you are unsure about a drug calculation or find that you cannot do the calculation, then the best course of action is to ask for help. Remember the rule: if in doubt, don't give it!

This is particularly important when nursing babies and children, where you have to take extra care with medications to ensure the correct dose is administered.

Critical reflection

Think about the following scenario: you are checking the medication record of a patient and see that a new order for digoxin has been prescribed. The order is for 62.5 mg. Would you give this dose?
- If yes, why? If no, why not? Where would you check for accuracy in this prescription?
- What are the potential outcomes of giving and not giving this medication?

Your responsibility as a student and registered nurse is to ensure that no harm comes to your patients because of your actions. In Australia, the system of measurement in healthcare is the metric system. You will have used this system of measurement as a student nurse in the practice setting, as well as having your knowledge and comprehension tested in examinations.

TABLE 9.1 METRIC MEASURES USED IN HEALTHCARE

WEIGHTS	VOLUME	LENGTH AND DEPTH
Kilograms	Litres	Kilometres
Grams	Millilitres	Metres
Milligrams		Centimetres

Critical reflection

List the areas in clinical practice where you would use the following measures and why:
- weight measures
- volume measures
- length or depth measures.

Literacy competencies

In the context of nursing practice, literacy skills are necessary for communication with patients, other health professionals and other workers in the healthcare organisation. Literacy skills include English language speaking skills and English language writing skills.

To provide safe, competent care to your patients, good literacy and language skills are essential. Communications relating to patient care will have to be understood by diverse groups of people whose first language may not be English and who may not have a clinical background. Accurate, well-written, and easily understood patient records promote seamless care, especially if patients are moved on to other healthcare teams. Accurate record keeping is important for nurses following you on a shift, and becomes more important if the next shift of nurses are agency or relief nurses, unfamiliar with the patients and their care needs.

You should know by now that an important aspect of being a registered nurse is writing and maintaining accurate patient records. As a student nurse, you will have written academic papers as assignments and will be marked down for poor use of language and grammatical inconsistencies.

All healthcare organisation and clinical units will have a standard format for entering information into the patient record. While in most organisations around the country the patient record is integrated, you may find yourself working in an organisation where the nursing information is kept separate from other health professionals. Logistically, this can be a problem, especially if you are trying to develop a plan of care or are changing an existing plan of care using a number of information sources. The patient record is also a legal document, so it is imperative that the nursing entries are accurate, easily understood and relevant. Where healthcare organisations are working with electronic patient records, well-written, succinct and current information from nurses is required, particularly if the model of care is multidisciplinary.

The patient record is a record of the patient's period in a hospital or healthcare organisation. It must:

• specify the reason(s) the patient was in the care of the organisation
• record the treatments or interventions the patient received and from whom (with legible signatures)
• contain relevant and factual information
• be legible (this includes the signatures of the people making the entries).

Effective literacy skills include good language and writing competencies. This not only includes having a good vocabulary and the ability to spell correctly, but also knowledge of the language used in the clinical unit you are working in.

As clinical practice becomes increasingly specialised, the language used in the units also begins to reflect the specialist clinical practices of units. Abbreviations should be used with caution, and you should only use the abbreviations that the healthcare organisation allows. While we may be living and working in a digital age, the use of text language is not appropriate for patient records. Effective literacy competencies are necessary irrespective of the way information is transmitted or relayed between health professionals.

Information technology competencies

Increasingly, the use of information technology by nurses and other health professionals is becoming more common in healthcare organisations. Information technology is used for managing nursing practice; for staffing; for entering patient data and, in some cases, for electronic patient records. Patient care is becoming more technologically sophisticated and your responsibility is to ensure that your information technology skills are at a level that ensures you are competent. You will have been developing some of these competencies throughout your undergraduate program.

Information technology refers to the machines (computers) and applications (software) that provide the infrastructure support for **information systems**. *Information systems* are integrated, complex automated systems that are networked through computers and used to support **information management**, data collection and decision-making. *Information management* is the collection, interpretation and storage of information for a particular purpose, which for nurses is patient care.

You may have been introduced to nursing clinical information systems during your clinical placements. These systems are used to support clinical decision-making, as well as measuring patient nursing needs. It is in your best interests to become adept at using these information systems.

INFORMATION SYSTEMS – The software and hardware used by a healthcare organisation to communicate and record details of activities related to patient care.

INFORMATION MANAGEMENT – The collection and analysis of patient-related information by health professionals to plan and provide care and services to patients.

Information management competencies

Information management is an integral component of nursing work, because information is provided by nurses to the healthcare team involved in caring for patients. Information comes from a number of different sources, including the patient, and you will have been made aware of this during your clinical placement.

One important source of information used by nurses is the handover sheet or 'cheat sheet'. As a nurse, you will enter relevant information about your group of patients at handover, prior to commencing your shift. Information technology enables clinicians to have 24-hour access to patient care information, thus facilitating timely treatment and care delivery for patients. Nurses in some parts of Australia are trialling point-of-care devices such as handheld tablets and other mobile devices to communicate with other health professionals and to record patient information, as well as to receive relevant information such as test results. Some state departments of health are trialling versions of the electronic patient record, and you may be a part of these trials in your state or territory. Attending the training workshops for this will be important, not only for your skill development but also for your professional development. Attendance at these training sessions is another entry in your professional portfolio. The advent of the iPad and similar devices is adding another dimension to electronic information management.

In some aged care facilities, nurses use mobile phones and SMS texting to contact and communicate with other staff members. In the contemporary health and aged care sectors, the use of information technologies for communicating and transmitting information is an important element of a nurse's information management competency set.

Biomedical technology competencies

You will have been exposed to patient care technologies during your student nurse program and will have noticed that these technologies are becoming increasingly sophisticated and are now an essential part of nursing practice. Developing skills in the use of biomedical technologies should be an integral part of your competency development and included in your professional portfolio. One thing you will need to know is what do to if the equipment fails or breaks down—who to call, what to do, how to keep the patient safe, and the procedures to implement while managing the patient during the time it takes to repair the equipment or change it over.

Conflict management competencies

Managing conflict in nursing is discussed in nursing management textbooks, but it is as a registered nurse that you will first be exposed to conflict situations during your work day. As a student nurse, you may have been exposed to, or observed conflicts in the clinical area, but it will be as a registered nurse that you have to take positive action to minimise the negative outcomes of conflict.

Conflicts may arise:
- between nurses (**intraprofessional conflict**)
- between different groups of health professionals (**interprofessional conflict**)
- between nurses and patients (nurse–patient conflict).

Conflict is a fact of life when you have people from various backgrounds and with different value and belief systems working together in fast-paced, complex

INTRAPROFES-
SIONAL CONFLICT –
Conflicts that occur
between members of
the same profession.

INTERPROFESSIONAL
CONFLICT – Conflicts
that occur between
members of different
health professions.

and high-stress environments. Conflict may be defined as 'real or perceived differences in goals, values, ideas, attitudes, beliefs or actions' (Sullivan & Garland 2010, p. 296). An area of conflict for the new graduate nurse may arise when you go to do a procedure as you were taught at university but a more experienced nurse comes along and tells you 'we don't do it that way; we do it this way'. So how do you manage this potential conflict situation? The main conflict responses (Sullivan & Garland 2010) are:

- *Competing*—an all-out effort to win, characterised by anger and aggression. Other competing behaviours include arguing, criticising, name calling and blaming others. This can be a form of bullying and intimidation.
- *Avoiding*—refusing to confront the situation and denying a conflict exists. Avoidance behaviours are characterised by doing nothing, fear of embarrassment, fear of consequences, fear of making things worse and a lack of assertiveness. Avoiding can be a part of bullying behaviours.
- *Accommodating*—yielding, giving up in favour of the other person. Sometimes this is the best option when a consequence can be advantageous in the future. The saying 'pick your battles' can apply here. Accommodating is often used with people who are more senior to you.
- *Compromising*—making a deal, meeting the other person midway—you give up something and they give up something. This strategy is sometimes held up as the best solution, but it can be unsatisfying because you can feel as if you have not really achieved an optimal outcome, and often the underlying reasons for the conflict are left unresolved.
- *Collaborating*—everyone involved in the conflict situation works together to achieve a mutually agreed upon solution, following discussion and sharing of insights, perspectives and available options, agreeing on the best option for all.

Conflict is context-dependent. The same strategy cannot be applied to every conflict situation. As individuals, we also develop our own responses to conflict situations. Research has shown that nurses tend to overuse avoidance and compromise strategies when dealing with conflict, and underuse the other three strategies (Sullivan & Garland 2010, p. 153).

Developing self-awareness of your conflict responses is an important aspect of your professional development as a registered nurse. Self-awareness will help you to manage your conflict responses in a rational and reasoned way. It is the difference between reacting to a situation and responding to a situation.

Critical reflection

Reflect on how you approach and manage conflict situations. Consider a personal situation or a situation you encountered while on a clinical placement, as an example. What were your responses in this situation?

- Discuss a conflict situation where you avoided all the issues. Why do you think you engaged in avoiding behaviour? What were your feelings at the time? What was the outcome at the time?
- Think of a recent situation (personal or professional) where you gave in to the other party. Why did you give in? (You wanted to be well thought of, you were developing relationships, it was not a battle you felt you had to win, or you had no choice?) What was the outcome of this and what were your feelings?
- Recall a time when you stood up for yourself, when you truly believed that your opinion and solution was the right one. What were your feelings at the time and why were you so intent on standing your ground? What behaviours did you use and what was the impact of this? What was the outcome for you and for the conflict?
- Recall a time when the conflict situation was so bad all you wanted to do was leave and never return. What was the result of your leaving? Was the situation resolved? Did you return and why?

(Adapted from Sullivan & Garland 2010)

In the scenarios you discussed in your study group, thinking critically and reflectively, together with discussing the issues, may provide you with strategies to help you deal with conflict that perhaps you had not considered before.

Management competencies

MANAGEMENT –
A series of processes comprising assessing, planning, directing, controlling and evaluating to achieve goals. For nurses, management achieves patient goals and outcomes.

You might throw up your hands in horror at the idea of **management** competencies. Surely you are a clinician, not a manager? Well, the truth is that even as a clinician you will use management skills and strategies to:

- manage your own workload—setting priorities and managing your time
- manage the workload on a shift
- organise patients for procedures, discharge and transfer to other units
- delegate functions to other staff
- make decisions
- communicate
- manage information.

All of the above activities are management functions that are a part of the clinician's role, and you will have engaged with some of these activities in your clinical placements. Next time you listen to a handover and fill out your handover sheet, think about what you are doing. You are setting priorities, determining your own workload needs, and developing time-management skills. You develop time-management skills so that you can deliver nursing care to patients in a timely and organised manner. You develop your communication skills so that you can pass on relevant information to other health professionals and, of course, to patients.

Another management competency you may not have considered is the ability to work in a team or with others. From your clinical placement experiences, you will have observed that in contemporary healthcare organisations, healthcare teams are multidisciplinary, working together to achieve positive health outcomes for patients and the organisation. Teamwork has been defined as 'cooperative efforts by members of a group or team to achieve a common goal' (Dwyer & Hopwood 2010, p. 223). Being an effective team member means that you are able to:

- work with others
- contribute to the goals of the team by demonstrating good clinical practice
- participate in team meetings by reporting and recording patients' clinical conditions and any changes that may occur, as well as any concerns patients may express
- act as an advocate for patients when necessary.

As a team member, you support other team members with workload management if this is necessary.

You should take the opportunity while on clinical placement to observe team leaders:

- allocating team members to patients
- ensuring each team member is aware of what they need to do
- liaising with nurse managers if workload issues arise during the shift
- managing the administrative tasks that need to be completed.

All of these tasks underpin the effective and efficient management of a team of people on a shift, and the team leader has to have enough information, for example, to allocate team members to patients. It would not be very efficient to allocate the most inexperienced nurse to the sickest patient.

THEORY TO PRACTICE

While on clinical placement you notice an experienced registered nurse ignore a patient who is trying to get her attention. The patient is aged 87 years and is recovering from surgery that required she have an indwelling catheter for a time, post operatively. It is clear to you that the patient is distressed so, even though the patient is not allocated to you, you go over to see what is going on. The patient has an indwelling catheter that has become disconnected, creating a wet bed and causing discomfort to the patient. Using the appropriate techniques you reconnect the catheter and note this in the patient record. Having done this, you tell the registered nurse what has happened and the actions taken by you, and you mention that you would like some help in changing the patient's sheets and their pyjamas or nightgown and giving them a sponge to refresh them.

The registered nurse becomes angry with you and accuses you of interfering with her patients by stepping outside your student role and saying that she would have gone to the patient eventually. You try to explain that the patient was uncomfortable and distressed. The registered nurse says she will report you for working outside your scope of practice. You finish your shift quite distressed.

You return for your shift the next day and check on the patient and her records and find that your entry had been removed and replaced by the registered nurse's notes which differ from yours.

You find out from colleagues that the patient's family had made a complaint against the registered nurse following her discharge from hospital. And that the Nurse Unit Manager is investigating the complaint and talking with staff present at the time of the incident.

Discussion Questions

1. What is your immediate reaction on learning about the complaint investigation?
2. Would you describe the registered nurse's behaviour as professional?
3. Were the initial actions of the nurse within the NMBA competency standards?
4. Should you have reported this behaviour at the time or were you afraid to because you still had six weeks of placement in this organisation?
5. Would you describe this as a conflict situation?

Other Nursing Competencies

The NMBA national competencies are the core competencies for all registered nurses in Australia. While it is important to develop all competencies, there are some competencies which are a priority. These are:

- assessment competencies
- communication competencies
- critical thinking competencies
- cultural competencies.

Assessment competencies

In the nursing process framework, the first function is assessment, and rightly so. The first thing you do as a nurse is to assess your patient or group of patients. Assessment is a process of observation, asking questions and making judgments that will lead to a care plan that meets a patient's care needs at the time of admission to your clinical unit. So how do you develop good assessment skills? Good assessment skills begin with:

- a good clinical knowledge base
- the ability to observe the patient and note their physical appearance and behaviour
- the ability to note any clinical symptoms and know what the symptoms indicate
- the ability to ask the patient the right questions and then to ask more probing questions should the initial responses indicate more information is required
- the ability to note the non-verbal cues the patient may be exhibiting; for example, the patient's body language may not reflect what he or she is saying
- the ability to document the assessment accurately.

Assessment is an ongoing process and you are continually assessing patients' conditions during the course of your shift or work day. You are assessing patients when giving medication, attending to a patient's personal hygiene; beginning to mobilise patients; taking observations such as blood pressure, pulse or respiration; or monitoring patients following an emergency event or after a fall. Any activity that engages you with a patient is an opportunity for assessment, and any deviation from what is the norm for a patient is documented, reported and recorded in the patient record. Even an unconscious patient requires continual assessment. For example, while attending to the personal hygiene needs of the unconscious patient, you will be assessing:

- respiratory pattern and deteriorating gas exchange
- any airway impairment—need to clear secretions
- impact of immobility
- pressure ulcers, skin tears
- response to tactile stimuli
- nutritional and hydration status
- any deterioration in neurological status
- any alteration in cardiac status.

From this, you can see why assessment is a core competency for nurses. Nurses spend more time with patients than other health professionals, and so opportunities for continual assessment are always present. As you become more experienced, assessing patients becomes something you do unconsciously, and your ability to respond to even the smallest changes in a patient's clinical condition may start to seem intuitive.

Critical reflection

Think about the following scenario. You are working in a respiratory unit and are asked to assess a new patient. During the assessment you observe the following:

- The patient is drowsy, agitated and in considerable distress.
- The patient has difficulty in responding to your questions, because they have to take a breath every few words.
- You count the patient's respiratory rate and find it is more than 48 breaths per minute.
- You observe a central cyanosis.
- You observe that the patient has peripheral oedema.
- The patient is tachycardic—pulse rate of 132/minute.
- The patient is hypertensive: 210/100 mmHg.

- What do these signs and symptoms indicate to you?
- What sort of clinical judgment will you make?
- Are there any tests that you believe should be done to validate your clinical judgment? Should you initiate any treatment?
- What would you document in the patient's record?
- What will the nursing care plan that you develop for this patient look like?

Communication competencies

COMMUNICATION —
The exchange of words, ideas, information through speech, writing, behaviours, facial expressions, tone of voice. Communication can occur at a number of levels but the two most common levels are verbal and non-verbal (Marquis Huston 2012).

Communication is one of the most fundamental human activities. It is a complex process used to pass on information, to influence, to teach and to show emotion (Sullivan & Garland 2010). Nurses need good communication skills to demonstrate knowledge and insights, to empathise, to manage conflict, to show trustworthiness and professional integrity, and to teach other nurses and patients. The purpose of communication is to arrive at a shared understanding of the message being sent and received. Communication is not just the sending of a message: it is also about careful listening and monitoring of responses. To be a good communicator, you not only have to have good language skills, but also good listening skills. You also need good assessment skills, because sometimes the real message is in the subtext that is observed through the other person's body language, tone, volume and inflection of voice. Observing body language is important when dealing with patients, because there are times when patients may be uncomfortable discussing with virtual strangers issues they consider personal or intimate. There are also times when patients play down their levels of pain because of some underlying fears they may not have expressed to you. If you are astute and paying close attention to what the patient is *not* saying by observing the patient's body language and listening to their tone of voice, you will be able to make a more informed assessment and clinical judgment of the patient's clinical status and need for nursing interventions.

In most healthcare organisations, critical clinical information is transferred or transmitted using the ISBAR tool. ISBAR is used to improve the safety and accuracy of transferred information between health professionals.

ISBAR is a mnemonic that stands for:

I= identity

S=situation

B=background

A= assessment

R= recommendation.

Further information about ISBAR may be found at: http://www.sahealth.sa.gov. au/wps/wcm/connect/public+content/sa+health+internet/clinical+resources/ safety+and+quality/clinical+handover/isbar+-+identify+situation+background+ assessment+and+recommendation.

Effective communicators have a well-developed vocabulary and know the words to use in any situation. This means that when you are talking with patients you do not use medical or nursing language, but instead speak to the patient in language they can understand. You also avoid distorting communication by using abbreviations that others do not understand. Because of the nature of their work, nurses sometimes use humour to defuse situations or debrief following a critical event. It is important to know that not everyone may share your humour, and others may find it offensive, so you need to be mindful of this. Also, nurses from other cultures may find it difficult to understand Australian slang; be mindful of this and use language that everyone can understand.

Feedback is another aspect of good communication, so it is important that you give feedback to anyone to whom you have delegated work. Feedback is not criticism or meant to be negative but should be an objective assessment of the outcomes of an event or intervention. For example, you may have participated in the emergency resuscitation of a patient in your unit. There was a successful outcome for the patient, but if this was your first emergency resuscitation then you would like to receive feedback about your involvement in the procedure, noting the good points and the areas in which you could improve. The emergency resuscitation event is one area where if the communication is not clear, succinct and to the point, outcomes can be less than optimal. The majority of healthcare organisations now offer debriefing sessions for staff following critical incidents or emergencies.

Critical reflection

As a student nurse on clinical placement, have you participated in an ISBAR handover?
- Were you able to identify the different elements of the ISBAR mnemonic during the handover?
- Do you believe the ISBAR communication tool supports the safety and accuracy of patient information?
- How confident are you in using the ISBAR tool?

Critical thinking competencies

CRITICAL THINKING — Complex thinking patterns that examine situations in terms of context and content. Critical thinkers also anticipate the consequences of decision-making.

This section discusses the concept of **critical thinking** in nursing and the relationship between critical thinking, nursing practice and patient outcomes. Critical thinking is an essential competency for you to develop if you are to become a safe, competent registered nurse. Critical thinking is a competency in the NMBA national competency standards for registered nurses (NMBA 2013). Critical thinking is 'purposeful and goal directed thinking' (Alfaro-LeFevre 2004, p. 4). The difference between critical thinking and thinking is that the former is purposeful, controlled and focused on achieving outcomes, while thinking can refer to any mental activity, including daydreaming or performing routine tasks (Alfaro-LeFevre 2004, p. 5).

Characteristics of a critical thinker

The characteristics of a critical thinker include:
- *being a lifelong learner*—for you, learning does not stop at graduation
- *being curious*—you continue to be curious about your work and your patients and ask why things occur
- *being confident*—you are confident in your ability to analyse questions or situations using inductive and deductive reasoning and to achieve the correct outcomes for patients
- *being courageous*—having the courage to challenge the status quo
- *being resilient*—not accepting setbacks, and persisting in finding the correct solutions
- *being self-aware*—having an awareness of your own limitations, knowing when to ask for help, and developing strategies to overcome these limitations
- working in groups.

Critical reflection

In your study group, discuss the characteristics of a critical thinker, and reflect on your critical thinking abilities. Reflect on times when you used critical thinking skills to achieve an outcome. How successful were you?

- Would you have done anything differently?
- Is there some attribute you would like to develop further?
- Did the clinical leaders you observed demonstrate critical thinking competencies?

Problem solving

Problem solving is another cognitive activity, different from critical thinking. To arrive at a solution in problem solving you:

- identify the problem or issue
- collect all the relevant information about the particular problem
- use the information to suggest several solutions
- make the best possible, safest decision based on the information you have at the time.

This last point is important, because to make the best possible decision you have to have knowledge of the context of the problem, knowledge of the patient and knowledge of the resources you have available to you. It is important to realise that a decision made for one patient may not necessarily be the best decision for another patient with a similar or the same problem or diagnosis. This is why it is important to have more than one solution, not discard any solutions, and to be able to apply a solution that meets the specific patient's needs. Problem solving is therefore context- and patient-dependent.

In nursing practice, the nursing process is a problem-solving process, made up of:

- assessment
- diagnosis
- planning
- implementation
- evaluation.

Critical reflection

Compare the nursing process with the clinical reasoning model presented below. Are there any similarities or differences? Apply each of these processes to the following scenario.

You have completed a physical assessment of a new patient, Mr W. You find that Mr W has pressure ulcers on his buttocks. The lesion on his left buttock is superficial and is located approximately 50 mm down the buttock next to the gluteal crease and measures 4 cm × 3 cm, with a depth of 0.2 cm. Mr W also has a sacral lesion with eschar present. You palpate the surrounding tissue and find that it is spongy to touch, with a smelly, purulent discharge. You ask Mr W whether these lesions are causing him any discomfort, and he replies 'no'. You report this to the team leader, who tells you to complete a care plan for Mr W and to take a swab from the wound.

- What do you do first? Why?
- Do you engage Mr W in developing his care plan?
- When developing the care plan, what risk factors will you need to consider? How will you determine the outcomes of care?

Clinical reasoning

Clinical reasoning is an important competency for nurses to develop. You will have developed some clinical reasoning ability from your study program, but ongoing development of this competency can be challenging. Levett-Jones et al. (2010) have developed a clinical reasoning model presented below. This model is based on 'five rights' of clinical reasoning. These 'five rights' are:

- Right cues—these are cues and groups of cues nurses observe while assessing a patient. These cues are identifiable psychosocial or physiological changes and form the basis for clinical reasoning.
- Right patient—this is the patient at risk of clinical deterioration. As a student nurse you need to learn how to recognise and prioritise patients at need of immediate care.
- Right time—this refers to the nurses' ability to recognise and act on the right cues appearing in a patient so the right nursing interventions can be implemented in a timely manner.
- Right action—this is a nursing action following a decision or clinical judgement. As student nurses you will need to learn how to synthesise patient clinical information to make the right clinical decisions from a number of suitable nursing interventions.
- Right reasons—the reasons have to be underpinned by accurate clinical assessments. (Levett-Jones et al. 2010, pp. 515–20).

Use this model to help you when you are on clinical placements and involved in the nursing care of acutely ill patients.

FIGURE 9.1 THE CLINICAL REASONING PROCESS WITH DESCRIPTORS

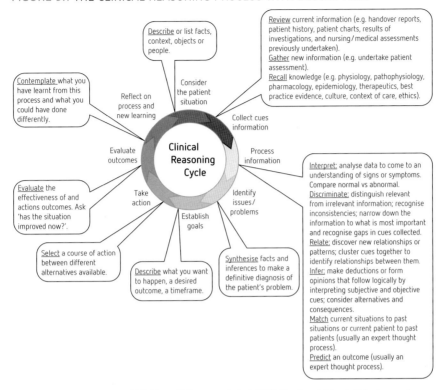

Source: Levett-Jones T, Hoffman K, Dempsey J et al. 2010, The five rights of clinical reasoning: an educational model to enhance nursing students ability to identify and manage clinically 'at risk' patients. *Nurse Education Today*, vol. 30 pp. 515–20.

THEORY TO PRACTICE

Non-English-speaking patient

Mr T, a 52-year-old man from a non-English-speaking background was admitted to the coronary care unit with acute heart failure. He had experienced chest pain two days prior to the admission but did not seek medical help. His family had administered traditional medicines in accordance with their cultural beliefs. Mr T had otherwise been a fit and healthy man with no other known medical problems.

On examination, Mr T was found to have left-sided heart failure and pulmonary oedema. His blood pressure was low (90/50) and his pulse 110. He was sweaty with cool peripheries. These signs were suggestive of cardiogenic shock.

His electrocardiograph (ECG) showed that he had a completed anterior myocardial infarction. A subsequent echocardiogram showed that Mr T had an ejection fraction of 21 per cent (normally, it is around 80 per cent), which meant that the left ventricle was severely impaired and could not maintain an adequate cardiac output, resulting in a backlog of fluid in the lungs and pulmonary oedema.

The normal treatment for acute myocardial infarction is reperfusion therapy (opening of the blocked coronary artery by thrombolytic 'clotbuster' drugs or balloon angioplasty). Unfortunately, Mr T presented to the hospital too late for this treatment, which needs to be administered within six hours of onset of the infarct for best results. He had already completed his infarct, and therefore the muscle supplied by the blocked artery was dead: therefore, there was nothing to be gained by opening the artery supplying this muscle.

Mr T was treated with IV medications to try and increase cardiac output and offload fluid to reduce the congestion on his lungs. However, in spite of best efforts, his blood pressure fell even further, his urine output decreased and his pulmonary oedema worsened.

Given these factors, the treating medical team decided that Mr T had a condition that was not reversible and that he should be given comfort care and not cardiopulmonary resuscitation (CPR) in the event of a cardiac arrest. However, all IV medication would be continued.

Mr T did not speak English, and nor did his wife and daughter, who were there with him. His son did speak English, however, and so the medical team explained the situation to the son and then left the son to explain the situation to the rest of his family and his father. The son agreed that all current efforts to help his father would continue, but in the event of cardiac arrest, he would not have CPR. The doctor wrote up IV Morphine 2.5–10 mg prn for comfort care.

In the setting of pulmonary oedema, morphine can reduce congestion in the pulmonary capillary beds, therefore it may have an alleviating effect. It also reduces pain and anxiety in patients. However, it may also result in respiratory depression which can, in the extreme, be fatal.

Shortly after the doctor had discussed the situation with the son, Mr T became extremely distressed and short of breath. The nurse listened to his lungs and could hear that he had fluid up to the apices (the entire lung field). His family were distraught, and through the son, requested that the nurse give him something to help him. The nurse drew up morphine, and considering the size of Mr T and his distress decided to give him 10 mg. She checked it with another registered nurse, as was policy for drug administration.

As the nurse finished administering the morphine, Mr T went into asystole (absence of heartbeat). Mr T stopped breathing and the monitor alarmed for asystole. The family all looked accusingly at the nurse.

Questions

1. Discuss the following questions about this case study in your study group.
2. How would you use the clinical reasoning model in this situation?
3. How helpful do you believe the model is?
4. Has using the model in this scenario helped you develop your clinical reasoning skills/competencies?

SUMMARY

This chapter is about the essential skills and competencies you will need to further develop as you move through your TPPP and beyond. The skills and competencies discussed in this chapter are fundamental for registered nurses working in contemporary healthcare environments. The twenty-first-century healthcare environment is technologically rich, with technologies changing at a fast pace. You have been introduced to a clinical reasoning model developed in Australia by Australian nurses.

All the skills and competencies listed in this chapter are underpinned by critical thinking skills, and the registered nurse of the twenty-first century is first and foremost a critical thinker. Effective critical thinking skills enable you to manage and disseminate information; enhance your information literacy skills; enhance your cultural competencies; and certainly enhance your clinical judgment and decision-making skills. Critical thinking is at the core of safe, competent nursing practice.

Discussion questions

1. In your opinion, what are the core competencies for nurses? Give reasons for your responses.
2. What is your understanding of clinical reasoning?
3. Identify the five rights of clinical reasoning in the case studies presented in this chapter.

Further Reading

Edwards A & Elwyn G 2009, *Shared decision making in health care*, 2nd edn, Oxford University Press UK, chapter 1.

Higgs, J, Jones MA, Loftus, S & Christensen, N 2008, *Clinical reasoning in the health professions*, 3rd edn, Butterworth Heinemann Elsevier, Philadelphia, pp. 3–101.

Melnyk, BM, Fineout-Overholt E 2011, *Evidence-based practice in nursing and healthcare*, 2nd edn, Wolters Kluwer/Lippincott Williams & Wilkins, chapters 1–4.

Windsor, C, Douglas, C & Harvey, T 2012, Nursing and competencies—a natural fit: the politics of skill/competency formation in nursing. *Nursing Inquiry* vol. 19(3), pp. 213–22.

Useful websites

Nursing and Midwifery Board of Australia. http://www.nursingmidwiferyboard.gov.au/

Competency development in the new registered nurse http://www.ncbi.nlm.nih.gov/pubmed/18323143

SA Health- ISBAR http://www.sahealth.sa.gov.au/wps/wcm/connect/public+content/sa+health+internet/clinical+resources/safety+and+quality/clinical+handover/isbar+-+identify+situation+background+assessment+and+recommendation

References

Alfaro-LeFevre, R 2009 *Critical thinking and clinical judgement*, 4th edn, Elsevier Science, USA.

Dwyer, J & Hopwood, N 2010 *Management strategies and skills*, McGraw-Hill, Australia.

Goleman, D 2005, *Emotional intelligence*, Bantam Books, New York.

Jordan, S 2011, 'Signposting the causes of medication errors', *International Nursing Review*, vol. 58, issue 1, pp. 45–6.

Levett-Jones, T, Hoffman, K, Dempsey, J, Yeun-Sim Jeong S, Noble, D, Norton CA, Roche, J & Hickey, N 2010, 'The five rights' of clinical reasoning: An educational model to enhance nursing students' ability to identify and manage clinically "at risk" patients', *Nurse Education Today*, vol. 30, pp. 515–20.

Marquis, BL & Huston, CJ 2012, *Leadership roles and management functions in nursing*, 7th edn, Wolters Kluwer Lippincott Williams and Wilkins, Philadelphia.

Sherwood, G 2012, 'Quality and safety: global issues and strategies', in G. Sherwood, J N Barnsteiner (Eds), *Quality and safety in nursing: a competency approach to improving outcomes*, John Wiley & Sons Inc., chapter 17.

Sullivan EJ and Garland G. 2010, *Practical leadership and management in nursing*, Pearson Education Limited, Harlow, Great Britain.

Translating Research Knowledge into Practice

10

ANNE HOFMEYER

LEARNING OBJECTIVES

After reading this chapter, you will be able to:

- explain why the translation of research knowledge and evidence into practice is needed to ensure safety and quality in health care
- discuss knowledge translation (KT), knowledge-to-action, and clinical decision-making
- outline the significance of building networks for KT
- identify the features and relevance of Integrated KT and End-of-Grant KT plans
- identify the features of well-written abstracts, presentations and articles
- outline a five-step guide to translate research evidence into practice.

KEY TERMS

End-of-grant knowledge translation plan
Evidence-based practice (EBP)
Evidence–practice gap
Integrated knowledge translation plan
Knowledge to action
Knowledge translation (KT)
Quality of care

Introduction

This chapter provides an overview of the importance of translation of research knowledge into clinical practice, and draws conceptual links with the knowledge translation and evidence-based practice literature. Interest in the literature has shifted from the synthesis of evidence to the translation of knowledge and implementation of relevant evidence into action to address the **evidence–practice gap**. The overarching aim to deliver best practices in health care is now focused on the complex process of implementing evidence from literature and guidelines at the 'point-of-care' in practice (Dogherty et al. 2013, p. 129). Delivering quality patient outcomes, informed by best evidence, is the foundational goal of every nurse.

EVIDENCE– PRACTICE GAP – The degree to which health services for individuals and populations increase the likelihood of desired health outcomes and are consistent with current professional knowledge.

The Nursing and Midwifery Board of Australia (2006) developed competency standards for the registered nurse specifying that nurses must demonstrate analytical skill in accessing and evaluating relevant forms of evidence and implementing this evidence in the provision of nursing care. Nurses are expected to locate, critically appraise, understand and apply research findings in their clinical practice (Crookes & Davies 2004, p. xii). However, in reality, this expectation creates a sense of 'deer in the headlights' for many nurses, causing them to feel uncertain about how to proceed (Gerrish et al. 2008; Fineout-Overholt & Johnston 2005a). We therefore present a five-step guide (Melnyk & Fineout-Overholt 2002) to help translate research knowledge into action, and to improve clinical practice and quality care for patients. The steps provide undergraduate nurses with a beginning understanding of this significant topic and a guide on how to demonstrate a degree of readiness to systematically respond and meet expectations.

What is the problem?

Landmark studies investigating the quality of health care in the USA and Netherlands reported that 'at least 30–40 per cent of patients do not receive health care according to current scientific evidence, while 20 per cent or more of care provided is not needed or potentially harmful to patients' (McGlynn et al. 2003; Grol & Grimshaw 2003). The translation and implementation (utilisation) of recommended scientific evidence into routine healthcare and policy decisions is haphazard, inconsistent and poorly coordinated (Eccles et al. 2005; McGlynn et al. 2003). Despite the existence of abundant clinical and health policy scientific evidence, gaps between best practice and actual clinical care persist, due to a widespread failure to implement scientific evidence (Straus et al. 2009; Grol & Wensing 2004). Therefore, a better understanding of the dynamics of the translation of research (use of evidence) into clinical decision-making practice is urgently needed, to improve relevant, effective and quality healthcare delivery. The US Institute of Medicine (IOM) analysed over 100 definitions of '**quality of care**' in healthcare services and developed a definition in 1990 that remains relevant in the twenty-first century:

> *Quality of care is the degree to which health services for individuals and populations increase the likelihood of desired health outcomes and are consistent with current professional knowledge. (IOM 1990, p. 21).*

Implicit in this definition is the expectation that healthcare professionals must use 'current professional knowledge' and research evidence in their decision-making. The IOM argues the healthcare system regularly harms patients and

QUALITY OF CARE – The degree to which health services for individuals and populations increase the likelihood of desired health outcomes and are consistent with current professional knowledge.

'routinely falls short in its ability to translate knowledge into practice and to apply new technology safely and appropriately' (IOM 2001). This gap (due to the slow implementation of evidence-based practice (EBP)) presents a major problem for managers, who have the responsibility to promote patient safety, research use in clinical decision-making and EBP in their organisations.

Likewise, in Australia, the safety and quality of health care is important to healthcare policy-makers, administrators, clinicians and the general public, so efforts to deliver this desired outcome continue. The National Health and Medical Research Council (NHMRC) CEO Warwick Anderson (2012) noted:

> The creation of knowledge through research underpins improvement in Australia's health service delivery and intervention. However, it is widely acknowledged that there is a gap between discovery and implementation of knowledge from research. This gap slows the uptake of the benefits from research, for patients and for the operation of the health system. Closing this gap is a daunting task exacerbated by the volume of research that is available and the need to sometimes change commonly accepted beliefs and behaviours.

Therefore, the goal is to bridge the **knowledge-to-action** gap to improve the timely access to relevant research knowledge, in order to facilitate its uptake to improve decision-making. Bridging the knowledge-to-action gap requires attitudinal and structural change (individual, organisational and system). Potential barriers (such as practice based on tradition) and incentives for achieving change in practice, and effective strategies to improve evidence-informed decision-making by clinicians need to be better understood. There is an urgent need for continuing education in EBP to be available for all nurses in clinical practice (Melnyk & Fineout-Overholt 2002).

KNOWLEDGE-TO-ACTION – The translation of research knowledge into clinical practice.

Critical reflection

Reflect on some of your previous clinical learning experiences from your nursing program.

- Describe a healthcare problem that arose during your placement. What happened?
- Explain the relevance of the problem, why it was important and to whom.
- Who was impacted by the problem?
- What solutions were implemented?
- What gaps remained?
- What knowledge or research evidence do you think is needed to address the gap in order to solve the problem?
- Draft a researchable question to investigate the problem.

ANNE HOFMEYER

What and who has to change?

Typically, the primary role of researchers has been the creation of knowledge and dissemination via traditional modes such as peer-reviewed journals and conference presentations. The new field of knowledge translation science developed about two decades ago in response to widespread global concerns about the haphazard implementation of research evidence in health care (Straus et al. 2009; Grol & Wensing 2004; Eccles et al. 2005; McGlynn et al. 2003). The responsibility is now on the researcher to change and to do more. Later in this chapter we will consider various formats to disseminate research knowledge to specific audiences, such as briefing reports, conference presentations, posters and refereed journal publications.

What is Knowledge Translation?

KNOWLEDGE TRANSLATION (KT) – The process of moving evidence into practice.

Knowledge translation (KT) can be understood as the science of methods to integrate and simplify knowledge into usable formats, and the study of potential barriers and enablers inherent in the process for organisations and individuals (Straus et al. 2009; Graham et al. 2006). KT refers to the assessment, review and implementation of scientific research evidence into practice. KT goes beyond traditional dissemination—it is an ongoing iterative process of engagement which is the best predictor for seeing the findings applied (Lomas 2000). This process takes place within a complex system of interactions between researchers and knowledge users which may vary in intensity, complexity and level of engagement, depending on the nature of the research and the findings, as well as the needs of the particular knowledge user.

KT is a *social process* that occurs within relationships and across professional networks (Estabrooks et al. 2006) and disciplinary and multidisciplinary teams (Hofmeyer & Cummings 2013). Knowledge is exchanged between people, so networks and norms (e.g. cooperation and trust) play a crucial role in facilitating learning and increased application of relevant knowledge.

An extensive review of the knowledge translation literature is beyond the scope and purpose of this chapter. There are numerous contributions to the knowledge translation and implementation science literature (for example: Estabrooks et al. 2006; Graham et al. 2006; Straus et al. 2009; Kitson, 2011). The purpose of this chapter is to provide a basic overview so nurses understand that KT is about moving research evidence and knowledge into action —closing the gap between *knowing* and *doing* to address the evidence–practice gap. Although there are various terms associated with this work, the goal is similar.

KT methods aim to close the knowledge-to-action gap (Straus et al. 2009; Graham et al. 2006). The focus is on the processes that influence *how* research knowledge is generated, communicated and used, as well as the potential barriers and incentives for achieving change in different contexts. Researchers and stakeholders collaborate to identify and solve everyday problems. KT is vital because, first, as studies have proven, the creation of new knowledge does not (on its own) lead to implementation or impacts on health. Second, researchers must demonstrate greater accountability for their funding from taxpayer dollars by doing more in terms of dissemination to ensure evidence is available for use in policy and practice. Bridging the 'evidence-to-practice' gap requires change at multiple levels (individual, organisational and system), so potential barriers and incentives for change need to be identified at each level. The mechanisms and strategies must be tailored to bring about change in specific organisational contexts and with different professional groups (Grol & Wensing 2004) in order to facilitate a patient-centred model of care.

Forms of evidence

A patient-centred model of care features the use of current evidence in decision-making by a range of healthcare professionals, and takes into account the preferences of the patient and family in the provision of best practice and, ultimately, quality care. Evidence can be derived from many sources, including research. We are reminded that a patient-centred model of care incorporates the knowledge and preferences of the patient in the decision-making. Rycroft-Malone and colleagues (2004, p. 81) 'outlines the potential contribution of four types of evidence in the delivery of care, namely research, clinical experience, patient experience and information from the local context'. The authors challenge nurses to incorporate several sources of knowledge into their clinical decision-making when planning quality care with patients and their families.

Dissemination of research evidence

Researchers must plan new approaches to ensure their research evidence is understood and accessible to inform policy and clinical decision-making. Increasingly, funding organisations are expecting researchers to include KT dissemination plans in grant proposals to facilitate the uptake of evidence. The onus is now on the researcher to 'translate' their research knowledge into plain language formats that are easily accessible and appropriate for those who might apply the knowledge. Such individuals are referred to as 'end users' or 'specific/desired audiences' in the literature. There are two main KT dissemination approaches

INTEGRATED KNOWLEDGE TRANSLATION PLAN – A plan in which potential users of the research knowledge are involved in the entire research process; that is, those who generate research knowledge and those who might use it (end users) work together to shape the research project within a collaborative relationship that is built on trust and cooperation.

END-OF-GRANT KNOWLEDGE TRANSLATION PLAN – The researcher develops and implements a plan for disseminating findings that includes traditional dissemination activities such as publications in peer-reviewed journals and conference presentations, and additional modes of dissemination.

to close the gap between *knowing* and *doing* (moving research knowledge into practice), **integrated knowledge translation plans** and **end-of-grant knowledge translation plans** (CIHR 2010; Lapaige 2010; Lomas 2000). Each approach has specific goals and suitability for different types of projects, so researchers need to ensure congruence.

Integrated knowledge translation plans

In integrated KT activities, potential users of the research knowledge are involved in the entire research process. This means that those who generate research knowledge and those who might use it (end users) work together to shape the research project within a collaborative relationship that is built on trust and cooperation. Individuals such as researchers, policy-makers, administrators, clinicians, consumers and stakeholders collaborate to determine the research questions and decide on the methodology. They are involved in data collection and tools development, interpreting findings and collaborating to disseminate the research results in relevant formats. This approach is similar to collaborative research, action-oriented research, and co-production of knowledge, and typically generates research findings that are more likely be relevant to, and used by the end users (CIHR 2010). A key element in the KT plan is the dissemination of findings in non-traditional formats, such as two-page summaries in plain language, video presentations, and fact sheets to explain how findings could be implemented in practice. So, when researchers present evidence in clear and accessible formats, they increase the likelihood that findings will be used in clinical decision-making. Integrated KT can be understood as both a process and the outcome (Lapaige 2010). It is about investing in collaborative relationships across sectors to ensure research questions are relevant, timely and generate accessible findings to address real-world problems.

End-of-grant knowledge translation plans

It is not always relevant or appropriate to incorporate an integrated KT dissemination plan into a project or involve various stakeholders throughout the life of the project. For this reason, researchers may plan to use 'end-of-grant' KT activities to disseminate findings to stakeholders when the project is completed. In 'end-of-grant' KT, the researcher develops and implements a plan for disseminating findings that includes traditional dissemination activities such as publications in peer-reviewed journals and conference presentations, and additional modes of dissemination. For example, actions to communicate messages that are tailored to specific audiences such as summary briefing reports for policy-makers, administrators and clinicians and short plain language interactive educational sessions for patients and carers (CIHR 2010).

Tailoring messages to different audiences

Researchers use various formats to disseminate research knowledge to specific audiences; for example, summary reports, abstracts, conference presentations, posters and peer-reviewed journal publications. It is crucial to identify your specific audience—who you want to target, influence and provide easy access to the evidence/knowledge. Knowing your target audience and where they access information will help you develop an effective dissemination plan to promote research utilisation, improve research impact and ensure that research findings reach the appropriate audiences (CIHR 2010). The importance of using a range of approaches to communicate information and evidence to others merits serious consideration. You have been accessing information from peer-reviewed journals during your undergraduate program. There are numerous peer-reviewed journals in nursing and other disciplines. Each journal has a website where you can access information about the editorial board, the journal's specific aims and scope, and guidelines for manuscript preparation and submission.

The abstract is the summary statement that you read to decide if the content of the article is relevant to your purpose and whether you will retrieve the article. When you have sourced peer-reviewed journals for information to prepare assignments, you have possibly judged the relevance of some articles based on abstracts alone. If you have attended conferences, you would have read the titles and abstracts of presentations when making decisions about which sessions to attend. You have been making these judgments and decisions throughout your undergraduate studies and will continue to do so as a registered nurse. Editors of peer-reviewed journals and conference organisers provide very specific instructions about developing abstracts and manuscripts for publication and presentation. Adhering to the specified format and word count, and avoiding unnecessary abbreviations and spelling errors are paramount to ensure abstracts are reviewed. Abstracts are usually written in the past tense because the research has been conducted in the past. Abstracts must present complex ideas in understandable formats for the reader (Coad & Devitt 2006; Happell 2007). Well-written titles and abstracts are crucial to fostering dissemination of knowledge. Consider:

- What you look for in an abstract?
- What features of an abstract would convince you to retrieve the article or attend the conference presentation?

During your studies, you will have been asked to present your work in tutorial groups or workshops. How did you feel about preparing and delivering your presentation? Did you feel confident about speaking to a group of people? Did you prepare PowerPoint slides to illustrate the main points of your verbal presentation?

ANNE HOFMEYER

You will be expected to communicate your ideas clearly, in a range of workplace situations such as clinical handovers and seminars, so building your confidence and skills are essential. Developing effective skills for communicating your ideas to others is dependent on meticulous attention to detail, planning, seeking feedback from others and practice (Hardicre, Coad & Devitt 2007). Although many experienced speakers still experience anxiety, most say that careful preparation and practice boosts their confidence to deliver their presentation. Practise so you are confident that you can deliver your talk within the allocated time, and leave time for questions and dialogue with the audience. Three elements of an effective presentation are:

1. Introduce your topic and tell your audience what you intend to speak about.
2. Deliver your talk, including your methods, results and conclusions.
3. Summarise the most important points of your lecture for your audience.
   When preparing PowerPoint slides for a verbal presentation:
- Number your slides.
- Avoid using unfamiliar abbreviations or expressions.
- A coloured background for your slides usually works better than black and white.
- Limit your use of colours and keep colours simple.
- Use few words and avoid sentences.
- Try not to have more than six bullet points on each slide.
- Only include text you plan to discuss.
- Use several slides if you need to cover a detailed topic that cannot fit onto one slide.
- If you must refer to a particular slide more than once during your presentation, use duplicates instead of trying to return to the original each time.
- Sometimes, graphs can be more potent tools than words.
  Presentation delivery recommendations include:
- Speak slowly and clearly, do not pace.
- Ensure your text is prepared specifically for your presentation.
- Find time before your presentation to acquaint yourself with the operation of the podium and location of equipment. Conference staff will be present to assist you.
- Speak in accordance with your slide sequence.
- Use a laser pointer to guide the audience. Do not wave the pointer around the slide.
- Stay within the time limit allocated for your presentation.
- Practise, practise, practise!

Consider rewriting your presentation for publication so you can reach a wider audience (Gross & Fonteyn 2008).

When designing a poster, consider its visual appeal and how it can best communicate knowledge to others (Miller 2007). Consider: who you want as your target audience for the poster content (e.g. policy-makers, hospital administrators, front-line managers, front-line nurses, other disciplines, patients and/or another group).

THEORY TO PRACTICE

You are meeting with nurses in your emergency department to design a discharge planning clinical project and a KT plan to investigate the increased frequency of visits by elderly patients with minor ailments to the department. You plan to disseminate findings to various stakeholders: patients and carers, other healthcare providers in the hospital, general practitioner (GP) services and community nurses who provide discharge care for your patients.

You have decided to use the *Knowledge Translation Planning Template-R* (TM) (Barwick 2013) to guide project planning with your team. The *Knowledge Translation Planning Template-R* (TM) was developed to create KT plans for research projects in all settings, and has been used in a variety of sectors (e.g. health, education, mental health). You can use the template, along with accompanying guides, to develop you own KT plan. Many funding bodies now require a plan to disseminate results, so this would be an excellent template to use to develop your plan. Access the *Knowledge Translation Planning Template-R* (TM) using the website address in the 'Useful websites' section at the end of this chapter.

Print the template and make a copy for each team member. The template can be used as a guide for discussion between team members, to plan and evaluate the steps in your KT strategy. Barriers to implementation of findings must be considered as well.

Discussion Questions

Thinking about your project:
1. Describe your target audience/s?
2. How would you develop a plan to disseminate and implement your findings so that they reach your target audience/s?
3. Ask all the team members to jot down their responses to the questions in the *Knowledge Translation Planning Template-R* that are relevant to your project (not every question will be relevant).
4. What else do you need to consider in implementing your findings?

ANNE HOFMEYER

What is Evidence-Based Practice?

In the Sicily Statement on EBP paper (Dawes et al. 2005, p. 1) it is stated:

> *Evidence-Based Practice (EBP) requires that decisions about health care are based on the best available, current, valid evidence. These decisions should be made by those receiving care, informed by the tacit and explicit knowledge of those providing care, within the context of available resources.*

Dawes et al. (2005, p. 4) propose a five-step model of EBP to teach healthcare professionals the process of EBP and to foster a 'critical attitude to their own practice and to evidence' in order to provide best practice. Specifically, the five steps to guide curricula are as follows:

1. translation of uncertainty to an answerable question
2. search for and retrieval of evidence
3. critical appraisal of evidence for validity, clinical relevance and applicability
4. application of appraised evidence to practice
5. evaluation of performance.

Why is EBP important?

EVIDENCE-BASED PRACTICE (EBP) – Requires that decisions about healthcare are based on the best available, current, valid evidence. These decisions should be made by those receiving care, informed by the tacit and explicit knowledge of those providing care, within the context of available resources.

The traditional approach to teaching research to nurses has focused on curricula incorporating research methods to generate primary evidence (Fineout-Overholt & Johnson 2005a). While this educational approach has some merit, it is increasingly apparent that all nurses are not well educated or prepared to provide **evidence-based practice** because 'the prevailing culture fosters practice based on tradition' (Fineout-Overholt & Johnson 2005a, p. 37). Further, nurses are not convinced of the relevance of research to their everyday clinical practice (Fineout-Overholt & Johnson 2005a). Education in EBP is increasingly important to prepare nurses to think systematically to identify problems and provide care informed by the best available evidence. However, there is an overwhelming amount of new information generated annually, monthly and even weekly. Nurses cannot read everything that is published in order to keep current.

Instead, EBP teaches healthcare professionals how to find 'best available, current, valid, and relevant evidence' to be used in decision-making (Dawes et al. 2005, p. 4). Nurses need to find reliable information in a systematic fashion and integrate with other forms of evidence/knowledge to provide best practice and quality patient outcomes (Fineout-Overholt & Johnson 2005a; Rycroft-Malone et al. 2004).

Step 0: Recognise uncertainty

Johnston and Fineout-Overholt (2005) have customised the EBP steps proposed by Dawes et al. (2005) for use in nursing education. They propose 'Step 0', a prerequisite to 'Step 1' of the EBP that focuses on developing an answerable question (Dawes et al. 2005). Step O is about clinicians and students developing skills to 'recognise and admit uncertainties' and doubts they may have in relation to their own knowledge and their practice (Johnston & Fineout-Overholt 2005). This recognition is the starting point to demonstrate a critical disposition toward one's own practice a degree of readiness to be a reflective practitioner committed to life-long learning and delivery of best practice. Critical reflection, discussion and inquiry between healthcare professionals supports this step of discernment and translating uncertainty into the formulation of a researchable question—Step1 (Johnston & Fineout-Overholt 2005; Dawes et al. 2005).

Step 1: Develop a researchable question

Guided critical reflection is the process used to identify a clinical problem that can then be developed into 'searchable, answerable clinical questions' (Fineout-Overholt & Johnston 2005b, p. 157). A standardised format is used to guide the process of formulating researchable questions. The PICOT framework can be used in the clinical setting or the classroom to guide this step. As described by Fineout-Overholt & Johnston (2005b, p. 158):

'P – Specific patient populations of interest,

I – Intervention of interest or issue of interest,

C – Comparison of interest (i.e. intervention or issue),

O – Outcome of interest,

T – Timeframe'.

The timeframe may not always be used, but is included in the PICOT format for consideration. Fineout-Overholt & Johnston (2005b, p. 158) suggest a clinical question can be generated through the following process:

- reflect on the clinical situation
- use a standardised format to formulate clinical questions
- use clinical question components to drive the search strategy
- determine the kind of evidence required to answer your clinical question
- identify the evaluation outcomes from the clinical question.

Fineout-Overholt & Johnston (2005b, p. 159) provide the following examples of different types of clinical questions using PICOT format and the types of evidence to answer the given question. Consider each example carefully.

TABLE 10.1 CLINICAL QUESTIONS USING PICOT FORMAT

QUESTIONS	TYPES OF EVIDENCE TO ANSWER THE QUESTION
Therapy: In patients living in a long-term care facility who are at risk for decubiti, what is the effect of an ongoing pressure ulcer prevention program compared to the standard of care (e.g. turning every two hours) on signs of emerging decubiti?	Randomised controlled trial (RCT)
Etiology: Are fair-skinned women who have prolonged unprotected UV ray exposure (>1 hour) at increased risk of melanoma compared to darker-skinned women without prolonged unprotected UV ray exposure?	Cohort study
Diagnosis or diagnostic test: Is d-dimer assay more accurate in diagnosing deep vein thrombosis compared to ultrasound?	RCT &/or Cohort Study
Prevention: For obese children, does the use of community recreation activities reduce the risk of diabetes mellitus compared to educational programs on lifestyle changes over a 6-month period?	Prospective study &/or RCT
Prognosis: Does dietary carbohydrate intake influence healthy weight maintenance (BMI <25) in patients who have family history of obesity (BMI >30)?	Cohort study &/or Case-Control Studies
Meaning: How do middle-aged women with fibromyalgia perceive loss of motor function?	Qualitative study

Critical reflection

Revisit the 'researchable question' that you developed earlier in this chapter to address a clinical problem you experienced during a clinical placement in your undergraduate nursing program. Consider the PICOT format and then carry out the following activity:

- Analyse your question to assess if all aspects of PICOT are included.
- Were any elements missing in your original researchable question?
- If yes, rewrite your question to address each element of PICOT.
- Explain how your researchable question has changed.
- Provide a rationale as to why you think the question is now more suitable to investigate as a clinical problem.
- What quality clinical outcomes are you aiming to achieve for patients?

This step to develop a researchable question is challenging and takes time. Hopefully, you will now appreciate why it is important to be confident that you are asking a relevant researchable question that will generate research evidence and provide the best answers for your clinical problem. Searching the literature requires key words to drive the search. The question you have generated using the PICOT format will provide the key words for your focused, systematic search of the databases and other repositories of research evidence.

Step 2: Search and retrieval

The second step in the EBP process is searching for suitable evidence to answer the clinical question (Fineout-Overholt et al. 2005). Gathering evidence requires competent skills in search techniques, access to electronic databases, libraries and expert librarians, and time available to undertake a systematic and thorough searching strategy. Many nurses have had little or no training to help them find dependable evidence to use in their practice (Pravikoff, Tanner & Pierce 2005). These factors are significant barriers to the implementation of EBP. Collaboration with others is essential for building techniques and effective skills in searching, determining levels of evidence (Levin & Chang 2014), and selecting the best available evidence to address the problem. Each element of the PICOT question provides key words, but must be combined with exclusion and inclusion criteria to narrow or explode the search to achieve a focused search strategy (Fineout-Overholt et al. 2005). Abstracts are first critiqued and, if assessed as relevant, the article is retrieved. Liaising with topic librarians who are familiar with your topic area is recommended to ensure this search step is conducted accurately and efficiently so that you find and retrieve relevant articles to answer the clinical question.

Step 3: Critical appraisal

The third step in the evidence-based practice (EBP) process is critical appraisal. Put simply: 'Critical appraisal is the process by which the practitioner evaluates research evidence in terms of (1) validity; (2) the results, i.e., the reliability; and (3) the applicability to practice' areas (Johnston & Fineout-Overholt 2006, p. 44). There are many tools, guides and checklists available to guide the process of critical appraisal, but all coalesce around the three areas that are applicable to both qualitative and quantitative studies. Teaching critical appraisal skills (CAS) is best learned with others first by conducting an appraisal of the evidence (e.g. peer-reviewed journal articles), second, by discussing the findings and then synthesising the evidence. Training through enacting CAS builds confidence and skills. Dawes et al. (2005, p. 5) believe an appraisal of the validity of a study and the importance of its outcomes will include the:

- suitability of the type of study to the type of question asked
- design of the study and sources of bias

- reliability of outcome measures chosen
- suitability and robustness of the analysis employed.

Notably, there is an expanding repository of clinical guidelines and resources that offer succinct summaries of research evidence for busy clinicians with little training in appraisal skills. While such resources serve a valuable purpose to bridge the evidence–practice gap, nurses still need to hone their critical appraisal skills to assess and synthesise research evidence and implement in individualised, patient-centred care to deliver quality patient outcomes.

Step 4: Implement evidence

The fourth step in the evidence-based practice (EBP) process is implementation (Fineout-Overholt & Johnston 2006). As researchers have shown, the translation and implementation (utilisation) of recommended scientific evidence into routine healthcare and policy decisions is haphazard, inconsistent, and poorly coordinated (Eccles et al. 2005; McGlynn et al. 2003). This means that problems in the healthcare system are not entirely about the need to conduct more research. Rather, they are about the implementation of what is already known (Fineout-Overholt & Johnston 2006). The process of implementation of EBP is complex and multifaceted, and potentially involves multiple organisational levels and stakeholders, other healthcare professionals, patients and carers. In order to successfully implement practice changes based on best evidence, it is essential to have the support of senior clinical managers. For example, if a different evidence-based wound care protocol is to be implemented, then the purchase of new wound care dressings and resources may need to be authorised by managers. In this way, building networks with others is a significant factor in translating knowledge and implementing new evidence in clinical practice, to deliver quality patient outcomes.

Step 5: Evaluation

To determine the success of the implementation of evidence into clinical practice, evaluation is step 5 in the EBP process (Fineout-Overholt & Johnston 2007). The overall goal is to implement evidence into practice, so evaluation of the outcome, for example, in terms of quality patient outcomes, is paramount. Nurses need to track and evaluate the effectiveness of their decision-making and practice by tracking the outcomes experienced by patients. A range of mechanisms and instruments are available to gather data (Fineout-Overholt & Johnston 2007). In summary, Fineout-Overholt and Johnston (2007, p. 56) specify that the key concepts in evaluation are:

- Healthcare decision-making must be data-driven
- Data must be accessible and user friendly to point of service providers

- Outcome evaluation must be interdisciplinary
- Outcome evaluation must be part of healthcare providers' curricula
- Healthcare education must engage in evaluating learners' integration of EBP.

The basic premise is that nurses and other healthcare professionals need to know whether they are successful in providing quality patient outcomes.

THEORY TO PRACTICE

Hannah Black is a 50-year old registered nurse in charge of a unit in an aged care facility in a large regional town. One of her patients, an 85-year old man with congestive cardiac disease and dementia, recently died from asphyxiation when his head became trapped between the side rails and the mattress on his bed. Hannah was taught during her nursing training to always ensure the side rails were up on patients' beds and she made sure the nurses who worked with her followed the same practice. On reflection, she wondered if that was the right approach to care for her patients. She asks several other nurses if they know what is considered best practice in this regard, but no one is able to provide relevant evidence. The practice of using side rails was longstanding in the unit and everyone followed the traditional practice/custom (without question) because they were taught to do it that way. Hannah has had little training to help her find new evidence, and the facility does not provide internet access for staff because the administration is concerned it might be used inappropriately. She has limited computer skills and uses the computer in the unit for patient care plans and internal email correspondence. Another barrier to EBP is that Hannah lacks confidence and doesn't know how to find information to establish if using side rails is the best intervention to keep patients with dementia safe in her unit.

You are a senior registered nurse and meet Hannah at a management training course in the city organised by the same aged care organisation. She tells you about what happened to the patient and how responsible she feels about the incident. She explains that she doesn't know how to access reliable evidence to solve the problem and to ensure best practice and care of patients in her unit long term. Adapted from Pravikoff et al. (2005).

Discussion Questions

Think about the problem and barriers that Hannah has shared with you.
1. How would you respond to Hannah?
2. What do you think is most important to consider?
3. List the elements of the problem.
4. What strategies would you recommend that Hannah could adopt to address barriers to EBP and to improve the situation?
5. What skills and resources do you think Hannah needs to access and develop?
6. Map out a plan of action for Hannah to implement to address the problem.
7. Develop a researchable question using PICOT.

SUMMARY

This chapter has provided you with introductory content about knowledge translation and various dissemination approaches, to facilitate the use of research knowledge by specific audiences to improve quality and safety in healthcare. You now have an appreciation of the different forms of knowledge to inform decision-making and patient-centred care and its significance. As a new registered nurse, you are also aware of your responsibility for ongoing learning and professional development, to be a competent user of research evidence and address the evidence–practice gap. The five-step process model of evidence-based practice (EBP) teaches nurses and other healthcare professionals the process of EBP, and fosters a critical attitude to their own practice and to evidence in order to provide best practice care. Nurses identify barriers to EBP as lack of time, and lack of searching skills and access to computers in work time. Change must occur at all levels of the healthcare system to address barriers in order to facilitate the use of relevant research evidence to reduce the evidence–practice gap and deliver quality, responsive healthcare. As Fineout-Overholt & Johnston (2006, p. 199) explain: 'In health care, we need to translate research into practice, value our clinical expertise and judgment, and include the patients' value and preferences in decision making; therefore, the major change for educators, clinical and academic, is to move in their own mind from evidence to action and mentor others to do the same'.

Discussion questions

1. How do you think the translation of research evidence into practice links with safety and quality in healthcare?

2. In addition to research knowledge or evidence generated from studies, what other forms of knowledge must be considered in clinical decision-making and why?

3. Identify an area of knowledge that you have gained during your studies at university which you were unable to transfer or implement during a clinical placement. Analyse the context and describe the barriers that prevented you from implementing the knowledge in your clinical decision-making and practice.

4. What challenges do you anticipate facing when promoting evidence-based practice in nursing? What strategies will you use to be successful in implementing the best available evidence?

5. Explain to another nurse the key reasons for promoting knowledge transfer and the uptake of research evidence in healthcare settings. How does that objective of improving the use of research evidence in decision-making link with calls for global change in healthcare quality and safety?

Further Reading

Straus, SE, Tetroe, J & Graham, I 2009, 'Defining knowledge translation', *Canadian Medical Association Journal*, vol. 181, no. 3–4, pp. 165–8.

Estabrooks, CA, Thompson, DS, Lovely, JJE & Hofmeyer, A 2006, 'A guide to knowledge translation theory', *Journal of Continuing Education in the Health Professions*, vol. 26, no. 1, pp. 25–36.

Graham, I, Logan, J, Harrison, M, Straus, S, Tetroe, J, Caswell, W & Robinson, N 2006, 'Lost in knowledge translation: Time for a map?', *The Journal of Continuing Education in the Health Professions*, vol. 36, no. 1. pp. 13–24.

Gerrish, K, Ashworth, P, Lacey, A & Bailey, J 2008, 'Developing evidence-based practice: experiences of senior and junior clinical nurses', *Journal of Advanced Nursing*, vol. 62, no. 1, pp. 62–73.

Levin, R & Chang, A 2014, 'Tactics for teaching evidence-based practice: determining level of evidence of a study', *Worldviews on Evidence-Based Nursing*, vol. 1, pp. 1–4.

Useful websites

Agency for Healthcare Research and Quality (AHRQ) Translating Research Into Practice (TRIP) Program: Initiative focusing on implementation techniques and factors associated with successfully translating research findings into diverse applied settings (http://www.ahrq.gov/research/trip2fac.htm).

Barwick, M (2013) 'Knowledge Translation Planning Template-R', Hospital for Sick Children Toronto, http://www.sickkidsfoundation.com/grants/knowledge.asp
http://www.sickkidsfoundation.com/grants/ktMethod/KT_Planning_Temp_Barwick.pdf
Knowledge Translation Planning Template

Campbell Collaboration (C2): International organisation that conducts systematic reviews of education, social welfare, social science research (http://www.campbellcollaboration.org).

Canadian Institute for Health Research (CIHR): Federal agency responsible for funding health research in Canada for KT research, development, and dissemination (http://www.cihr-irsc.gc.ca/e/29529.html).

Cochrane Collaboration: International organisation that conducts systematic reviews of health and medical research (http://www.cochrane.org).

The Australian Government has funded the work of the Cochrane Collaboration in Australia through the National Health and Medical Research Council since 2001. Through a funded five-year agreement to 2017 the NHMRC has ensured access to the Cochrane Library. The Cochrane Library can be accessed at www.thecochranelibrary.com and access is free to all residents of Australia.

Systematic reviews www.cochrane.org/cochrane-reviews.

Public Health Group http://ph.cochrane.org/.

Database of Abstracts of Reviews of Effects (DARE) http://onlinelibrary.wiley.com/o/cochrane/cochrane_cldare_articles_fs.html.

Knowledge Translation Program (KTP) University of Toronto, Canada: Multidisciplinary academic program developed to address the gap between research evidence and clinical practice and the need to focus on the processes through which knowledge is effectively translated into changed practices (http://www.stmichaelshospital.com/research/kt.php).

Knowledge Utilization Studies Program, University of Alberta, Canada: Focus on nursing, social sciences, and research utilization in nursing (http://www.kusp.ualberta.ca).

National Health Service (NHS) Centre for Reviews and Dissemination, University of York: Conducts systematic reviews of research and disseminates research-based information about the effects of interventions used in health and social care in UK (http://www.york.ac.uk/inst/crd/welcome.htm).

Evidence-based websites

Academic Center for Evidence Based Practice. University of Texas (http://www.acestar.uthscsa.edu/)— to advance evidence-based nursing practice, research, and education within an interdisciplinary context.

Evidence Based Nursing (http://ktclearinghouse.ca/cebm/syllabi/nursing). Centre for Evidence-Based Medicine, Toronto, Canada.

Nursing Knowledge International (http://www.nursingknowledge.org/Portal/main.aspx). Evidence-based content: Sigma Theta Tau International.

National Collaborating Centre for Methods and Tools. *Knowledge translation planning tool.* Hamilton, ON: McMaster University. http://www.nccmt.ca/registry/view/eng/131.html.

University of Minnesota, tutorials to describe evidence-based practice (www.lib.umn.edu/apps/instruction/ebp/)

References

Anderson, W 2012, 'New approach to identifying evidence–practice gaps and research priorities', NHMRC Research Translation Faculty. Media Release. NHMRC 17 August (https://www.nhmrc.gov.au/_files_nhmrc/media_releases/release_120817_rtf.pdf).

Barwick, M 2013, *Knowledge Translation Planning Template-R*, Hospital for Sick Children Toronto, www.melaniebarwick.com/training.php.

CIHR 2010, *More about Knowledge Translation.* Ottawa, ON: Canadian Institutes of Health Research http://www.cihr-irsc.gc.ca/e/39033.html accessed 18 February 2014.

Canadian Foundation for Healthcare Improvement (CFHI): http://www.cfhi-fcass.ca/Home.aspx.

Coad, J & Devitt, P (2006) ' Research dissemination: The art of writing an abstract for conferences', *Nurse Education in Practice*, vol. 6, no. 2, pp. 112–16.

Cook, DJ, Jaeschke, R & Guyatt, GH 1992, 'Critical appraisal of therapeutic interventions in the intensive care unit: human monoclonal antibody treatment in sepsis', *Journal of Intensive Care Medicine* vol. 7, no. 6, pp. 275–82.

Crookes, P & Davies, S (eds) 2004, *Research into practice: essential skills for reading and applying research in nursing and health care*, Baillière Tindall, Edinburgh.

Dawes, M, Summerskill, W, Glasziou, P, Cartabellotta, A, Martin, J, Hopayian, K, Porzsolt, F, Burls, A & Osborne, J 2005, 'Sicily statement on evidence-based practice', *BMC Medical Education* vol 5 (1). doi:10.1186/1472-6920-5-1.

Dogherty, E, Harrison, M, Graham, I, Vandyk, A & Keeping-Burke, L 2013, 'Turning knowledge into action at the point-of-care: the collective experiment of nurses facilitating the implementation of evidence-based practice', *Worldviews on Evidence-Based Nursing*, vol. 10, no. 3, pp 129–30.

Eccles, M, Grimshaw J, Walker, A, Johnston, M & Pitts, N 2005, 'Changing the behavior of healthcare professionals: the use of theory in promoting the uptake of research findings', *Journal Clinical Epidemiology*, vol. 58, no. 2, pp. 107–12.

Estabrooks, CA, Thompson, DS, Lovely, JJE & Hofmeyer, A 2006, 'A guide to knowledge translation theory', *Journal of Continuing Education in the Health Professions*, vol. 26, no. 1 pp. 25–36.

Fineout-Overholt, E & Johnston, L 2005a 'Teaching EBP: a challenge for educators in the 21st century', *Worldviews on Evidence-Based Nursing*, vol. 2, no. 1, pp. 37–9.

Fineout-Overholt, E & Johnston, L 2005b, 'Teaching EBP: asking searchable, answerable clinical questions', *Worldviews on Evidence-Based Nursing*, vol. 2, no. 3, pp. 157–60.

Fineout-Overholt, E & Johnston, L 2006, 'Teaching EBP: Implementation of evidence: moving from evidence to action', *Worldviews on Evidence-Based Nursing*, vol. 3, no. 4, pp. 194–200.

Fineout-Overholt, E & Johnston, L 2007, 'Evaluation: An essential step to the EBP process', *Worldviews on Evidence-Based Nursing'*, vol. 4, no. 1, pp. 54–9.

Fineout-Overholt, E, Hofstetter, S, Shell, L & Johnston, L 2005, 'Teaching EBP: getting to the gold: how to search for the best evidence', *Worldviews on Evidence-Based Nursing*, vol. 2, no. 4, pp. 207–11.

Gerrish, K, Ashworth, P, Lacey, A & Bailey, J 2008 'Developing evidence-based practice: experiences of senior and junior clinical nurses', *Journal of Advanced Nursing*, vol. 62, no. 1, pp. 62–73.

Graham, I, Logan, J, Harrison, M, Straus, S, Tetroe, J, Caswell, W & Robinson, N 2006, 'Lost in knowledge translation: time for a map?', *The Journal of Continuing Education in the Health Professions*, vol. 36, no. 1. pp. 13–24.

Grol, R & Wensing, M 2004, 'What drives changes? Barriers to and incentives for achieving evidence based practice', *Medical Journal of Australia*, vol. 1806, no. 6, pp. S57–S60.

Grol, R & Grimshaw, J 2003, 'From best evidence to best practice: effective implementation of change in patients' care'. *Lancet*, vol. 362, no. 9391, pp. 1225–30.

Gross, A & Fonteyn, M 2008, 'Turn your presentation into a published manuscript: advance evidence-based practice with a few simple steps,' *American Journal of Nursing*, vol. 108, no. 10, pp. 85–7.

Happell, B 2007, 'A no tears approach to writing an abstract for a conference presentation', *International Journal of Mental Health Nursing*, vol. 16, no. 6, pp. 447–52.

Hardicre, J, Coad, J & Devitt, P 2007, 'Ten steps to successful conference presentations', *British Journal of Nursing*, vol. 16, no. 7, pp. 402–4.

Hofmeyer, A & Cummings, G 2013, 'Working in multidisciplinary healthcare teams', in J Daly, S Speedy & D Jackson. (Eds), *Contexts of nursing*, 4th edn, Churchill Livingstone Elsevier, chapter 15, pp 253–70.

Institute of Medicine [IOM] (1990) *A strategy for quality assurance*, National Academy Press, Washington, DC.

Institute of Medicine [IOM] (2001) *Crossing the quality chasm: a new health system for the 21st century*, National Academy Press, Washington, DC.

Johnston, L & Fineout-Overholt, E 2005, 'Teaching EBP: getting from zero to one. Moving from recognizing and admitting uncertainties to asking searchable, answerable questions', *Worldviews on Evidence-Based Nursing*, vol. 2, no. 2, pp. 98–102.

Johnston, L & Fineout-Overholt, E 2006, 'Teaching EBP: the critical step of critically appraising the literature', *Worldviews on Evidence-Based Nursing*, vol. 1, no. 2, pp. 44–6.

Kitson, A 2011, 'Mechanics of knowledge translation', *International Journal of Evidence-Based Healthcare*, vol. 9, no. 2, pp. 79–80.

Lapaige, V 2010, Integrated knowledge translation for globally oriented public health practitioners and scientists: Framing together a sustainable transfrontier knowledge translation vision. *Journal of Multidisciplinary Healthcare*, vol. 3, no. 3, pp. 33–47.

Levin, R & Chang, A 2014, 'Tactics for teaching evidence-based practice: determining level of evidence of a study', *Worldviews on Evidence-Based Nursing*, vol.1, pp. 1–4.

Lomas, J 2000, 'Using linkage and exchange to move research into policy at a Canadian Foundation' *Health Affairs*, vol. 19, no. 3, pp. 236–40.

McGlynn, EA, Asch, SM & Adams, J 2003, 'The quality of health care delivered to adults in the United States', *New England Journal of Medicine*, vol. 348, no. 26, pp. 2635–45.

Melnyk, B & Fineout-Overholt, E 2002, 'Putting research into practice', *Reflections on Leadership*, vol. 28, no. 2, pp. 22–5, 45.

Miller, JE 2007, 'Preparing and presenting effective research posters', *Health Services Research*, vol. 42, (1 Pt 1), pp. 311–28, http://www.ncbi.nlm.nih.gov/pmc/articles/PMC1955747/.

Nursing and Midwifery Board of Australia 2006, *National competency standards for the registered nurse*, Nursing and Midwifery Board of Australia, Victoria, http://www.nursingmidwiferyboard.gov.au/Codes-Guidelines-Statements/Codes-Guidelines.aspx, accessed 5 February 2014.

Pravikoff, D, Tanner, A & Pierce, S 2005, 'Readiness of US nurses for evidence-based practice', *American Journal of Nursing*, vol. 105, no. 9, pp. 40–51.

Rycroft-Malone, J, Seer, K, Titchen, A, Harvey, G, Kitson, A & McCormack, B 2004, 'What counts as evidence in evidence-based practice?', *Journal of Advanced Nursing*, vol. 47, no. 1, pp. 81–90.

Straus, SE, Tetroe, J & Graham, I 2009, 'Defining knowledge translation', *Canadian Medical Association Journal*, vol. 181, no. 3-4, pp. 165–8.

Safety, Quality and the Registered Nurse

11

MARIA FEDORUK

LEARNING OBJECTIVES

After reading this chapter, you will be able to:

- demonstrate an understanding of the principles of risk management

- develop plans and strategies to ensure the safety of patients

- examine the factors affecting safety in the healthcare workplace

- measure the quality of nursing care provided

- understand the role of the registered nurse in clinical governance.

KEY TERMS

Accreditation
Australian Commission on Safety and Quality in Health Care (ACSQHC)
Clinical governance
Horizontal violence
National Safety and Quality Health Services Standards (NSQHSS)
Quality nursing practice
Risk management
Safe nursing practice
Workplace Health and Safety (WHS)

Introduction

This chapter introduces you to the role of the registered nurse in managing safety in the workplace. All nurses have a responsibility to deliver safe, competent nursing care to patients by working to established national standards of professional practice. There are two sets of standards for registered nurses in Australia. The Nursing and Midwifery Board of Australia (NMBA) provides registration standards (http://www.nursingmidwiferyboard.gov.au/Registration-Standards. aspx) and competency standards. (http://www.nursingmidwiferyboard.gov.au/ Codes-Guidelines-Statements/Codes-Guidelines.aspx).

The NMBA carries out functions as set by the *The Health Practitioner Regulation National Law Act*, in force in each state and territory (the National Law). Under the National Law the National Board has the power to register students. This regulatory approach is enshrined in legislation and has been implemented as a mechanism to protect the public (NMBA 2013). So you can see that safety and quality begin with your registration with the National Board.

Safety, Quality and the Registered Nurse

While on clinical placements you will have noticed the policies, procedures and clinical protocols used by healthcare professionals in the provision of care. These policies, procedures and protocols are based on evidence derived from research and are there to minimise risk to patients and staff.

In Australia, there is a national approach to managing safety and quality in healthcare using the **National Safety and Quality Health Service Standards (NSQHSS)** developed by the **Australian Commission on Safety and Quality in Health Care (ACSQHC)**. The ACSQHC is the peak body for managing safety and quality in health care through an **accreditation** process. Further information on the ACSQHC and the NSQHSS can be found at ACSQHC's website (http://www.safetyandquality.gov.au/our-work/national-standards-and-accreditation/).

Figure 11.1 provides a list of the NSQHSS standards used during accreditation.

FIGURE 11.1 NSQHSS STANDARDS

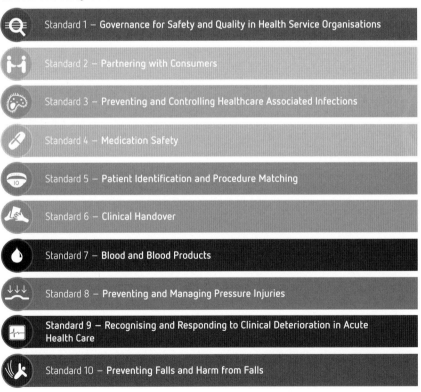

Standard 1 – Governance for Safety and Quality in Health Service Organisations

Standard 2 – Partnering with Consumers

Standard 3 – Preventing and Controlling Healthcare Associated Infections

Standard 4 – Medication Safety

Standard 5 – Patient Identification and Procedure Matching

Standard 6 – Clinical Handover

Standard 7 – Blood and Blood Products

Standard 8 – Preventing and Managing Pressure Injuries

Standard 9 – Recognising and Responding to Clinical Deterioration in Acute Health Care

Standard 10 – Preventing Falls and Harm from Falls

Source: ACSQHC 2012.

Critical reflection

In your study group or tutorial, read through the NSQHSS and see how they relate to your practice. Take the time to read through the criteria for each standard, and note how specific they are and how they relate to your practice.

Where do you think you will find a link between the registration standards and the NSQHSS?

An example of the national approach to managing risk in the healthcare workplace is the National Hand Hygiene Initiative (NHHI), organised by Hand Hygiene Australia. The purpose of the National Hand Hygiene Initiative is 'to develop a national approach to improving HH [hand hygiene] and monitor its effectiveness. This initiative is based on the World Health Organization (WHO) World Alliance for Patient Safety campaign (Hand Hygiene Australia 2011).

Other examples of national approaches to managing safety, quality and risk in healthcare include those noted by ACSQHC:

- national inpatient medication chart
- Australian safety and quality goals for healthcare
- national recommendations for user-applied labelling of injectable medicines, fluids and lines.

The World Health Organization (WHO) educational materials relating to patient safety and quality at an international level can be found on the WHO's website   (http://www.who.int/patientsafety/education/curriculum/Curriculum_ Tools/en/index1.html).

Inherent in this definition of **quality nursing practice** is that it is based on current knowledge that nurses access as part of their assessment and care planning processes. Therefore, it should be clear to you that the use of research-based evidence to inform your nursing practice is an integral component of the quality and safety elements of health services delivery in Australia.

In Australia, the conceptual framework for managing quality in health and nursing care is the Australian Safety and Quality Framework for Health Care (ACSQHC 2010). The three pillars of this framework are shown in figure 11.2.

QUALITY NURSING PRACTICE – Nursing practice that is competency-based on national standards, where patient outcomes exceed expectations. Data derived from research is used to inform nurses' practice.

SAFE NURSING PRACTICE – Nursing practice that is delivered as per standards-based clinical protocols and does not harm the patient.

FIGURE 11.2 THREE PILLARS OF THE AUSTRALIAN SAFETY AND QUALITY FRAMEWORK FOR HEALTH CARE

Safe, high-quality health is always:	What it means for me as a consumer or patient:	Areas for action by people in the health system:
1 CONSUMER CENTRED This means: Providing care that is easy for patients to get when they need it. Making sure that healthcare staff respect and respond to patient choices, needs and values. Forming partnerships between patients, their family, carers and healthcare providers.	I can get high-quality care when I need it. I have information I can understand. It helps me to make decisions about my health care. I can help to make my care safe. My health care is well organised. The doctors, nurses and managers all work together. I feel safe and well cared for. I know my healthcare rights. If something goes wrong, my healthcare team look after me. I receive an apology and a full explanation of what happened.	1.1 Develop method and models to help patients get health services when they need them. 1.2 Increase health literacy. 1.3 Partner with consumers, patients, families and carers to share decision making about their care. 1.4 Provide care that respects and is sensitive to different cultures. 1.5 Involve consumers, patients and carers in planning for safety and quality. 1.6 Improve continuity of care. 1.7 Minimise risks at handover. 1.8 Promote healthcare rights. 1.9 If something goes wrong, openly inform and support the patient.
2 DRIVEN BY INFORMATION This means: Using up-to-date knowledge and evidence to guide decisions about care. Safety and quality data are collected, analysed and fed back for improvement. Taking action to improve patients' experiences.	My care is based on the best knowledge and evidence. The outcome of my treatment and my experiences are used to help improve care.	2.1 Use agreed guidelines to reduce inappropriate variation in the delivery of care. 2.2 Collect and analyse safety and quality data to improve care. 2.3 Learn from patients' and carers' experiences. 2.4 Encourage and apply research that will improve safety and quality.
3 ORGANISED FOR SAFETY This means making safety a central feature of how healthcare facilities are run, how staff work and how funding is organised.	I know that the healthcare team, managers and governments all take my safety seriously. The health system is designed to provide safe, high-quality care for me, my family and my carers. When something goes wrong, actions are taken to prevent it happening to someone else.	3.1 Health staff take action for safety. 3.2 Health professionals take action for safety. 3.3 Managers and clinical leaders take action for safety. 3.4 Governments take action for safety. 3.5 Ensure funding models are designed to support safety and quality. 3.6 Support, implement and evaluate e-health. 3.7 Design and operate facilities, equipment and work processes for safety. 3.8 Take action to prevent or minimise harm from healthcare errors.

Source: ACSQHC 2010

While this framework takes a systems approach, you can see where nursing practice at the unit level fits. You can find more information relating to Australian Safety and Quality Framework for Health Care at http://www.safetyandquality.gov.au/wp-content/uploads/2011/01/ASQFHC-Guide-Healthcare-team.pdf.

This URL will take you to an ACSQHC document, 'Putting the framework into action' (ACSQHC 2010). You should have deduced by now that, in Australia, safety and quality are inextricably linked and, as the literature shows, nurses are important to the management of safety and quality in the healthcare sector. Even beginning registered nurses have a signifcant role in delivering safe, quality nursing care.

However, there is a downside to the provision of safe, quality nursing care. It is described in the literature as 'missed episodes of care' or errors of omission (Kalisch et al. 2009; Ball et al. 2014; Wakefield, 2014). Errors of omission are those related to missed aspects of nursing care which can result in negative outcomes for patients. Kalisch et al. (2009) differentiate between errors of omission and errors of commission, an example of the latter being administering the incorrect medication. Errors of omission involve not doing the right thing, such as turning a patient or not checking wound sites and intravenous sites. Both error types can result in adverse outcomes for patients and will be reported through the organisational incident reporting system.

Risk management

As a part of their quality and safety programs, all healthcare organisations now use a risk management matrix to support their risk management activities. There are five basic principles of **risk management**:

- Avoid risk
- Identify risk
- Analyse risk
- Evaluate risk
- Treat risks.

(ACSQHC 2013, p.2)

RISK MANAGEMENT — A program designed to identify, minimise and avoid risks to patients, staff, volunteers, visitors and all people who come into a healthcare organisation.

Figure 11.3 shows an example of a risk management matrix used for aseptic technique. This comes from the ACSQHS (2013). You can see how the separate factors can be assessed and scored separately. It is important to note that failure to identify potential sources of risk while caring for patients can result in adverse outcomes for patients.

Assessing risk is not confined to the clinical context only. As a registered nurse you will have to assess the physical environment for hazards to prevent trips and falls for staff and patients, and ensure that all safety precautions for individual patients have been established. An important aspect of safety and risk management is knowing what to do in emergencies, where patients and staff may have to be evacuated because of fires, bomb threats or any threat to the organisation that may harm patients, staff visitors volunteers.

FIGURE 11.3 EXAMPLE OF A RISK MANAGEMENT MATRIX USED FOR ASEPTIC TECHNIQUE

1. Clinical context			
Frequency	Controlled	Semi-controlled	Uncontrolled
Infrequent	1 = Low	4 = Low	6 = Medium
Occasional	4 = Low	6 = Medium	8 = High
Frequent	6 = Medium	8 = High	10 = Very high

2. Treatment type			
Frequency	Simple procedure	Complex procedure	Invasive procedure
Infrequent	1 = Low	4 = Low	6 = Medium
Occasional	4 = Low	6 = Medium	8 = High
Frequent	6 = Medium	8 = High	10 = Very high

3. Assessment of skills in aseptic technique			
Recent	Recent but changed clinical context	Assessed 1-3 years	Assessment unknown of >3 years
1 = Low	4 = Medium	4 = Medium	8 = High

Source ACSQHC (2013).

Minimising risk in the healthcare workplace is the responsibility of all health professionals—clinicians and non-clinicians. The organisation has a responsibility to provide workers with a safe working environment that includes:

- sufficient space to deliver patient care
- a hazard-free environment that will prevent injury to patients, staff and visitors
- equipment that is fully functional and well maintained
- a risk management program that is supported by policies, procedures and protocols
- education for staff relating to safety in the workplace, including emergency procedures (clinical and non-clinical)
- safe systems of work for all staff
- a system for reporting faults, for example, faulty equipment, environmental hazards, clinical errors
- a system for monitoring and evaluating the effectiveness of risk management strategies.

As a health professional, you also have responsibilities in relation to risk management. These include:

- working within your scope of practice (check the NMBA competencies for registered nurses and midwives)
- having the knowledge and competencies to work in the healthcare environment
- being able to respond appropriately in emergency situations
- knowing how to report faults in the workplace
- understanding your statutory obligations in relation to delivering safe patient care.

Clinical governance

Clinical governance is the term now being used to explain the systems used by healthcare organisations to ensure safety, quality and risk management in service delivery. Clinical governance is an umbrella term covering these elements. Governance of a health care organisation refers to the set of relationships established by a health service organisation between its executive, workforce and stakeholders links.

Governance provides the infrastructure support (policies, legislative frameworks, systems of work, resources and protocols) by which the organisation can achieve its corporate objectives.

It is important not to use these terms interchangeably.

CLINICAL GOVERNANCE – A system through which healthcare organisations are accountable for continuously improving the quality of their services and safeguarding standards of care.

The healthcare environment

Registered nurses have a pivotal role in managing safety in the healthcare environment, which includes ensuring a safe physical environment, ensuring compliance with established safe systems of work and reporting any risks identified when at work.

The healthcare environment for beginning registered nurses and, indeed, all nurses and healthcare workers, is both complex and dynamic. It can range from a clinical unit in a tertiary-level teaching hospital to a country hospital providing secondary health services and/or community services, or a stand-alone community service, providing community nursing and other health services. In the community-based setting, a nurse's work environment may include the car and the patient's home. A safe working environment for nurses can vary and be dependent on the location for nursing practice.

Because nurses work in diverse environments, ensuring a safe working environment can be problematic, especially in circumstances where the employer and the employee have no control over the site of nursing care. Nurses need to be aware of the policies and procedures relating to safe practice in their organisations, including the responsibilities of their employer, as well as their responsibilities as an employee under the **Workplace Health and Safety (WHS)** legislation in their state or territory. Inherent in the notion of safe nursing practice is that nurses are accountable for ensuring that their work practices comply with the legislation.

It should also be noted that work practices may legitimately vary because of differences in work environments and the availability of resources. For example, workplace safety in a tertiary-level teaching hospital may be defined differently to workplace safety for those working in the community. The core principles and the spirit of the legislation remain the same but the application of these principles is context-dependent.

Sources of error in the healthcare workplace

In healthcare organisations in developed countries, there are seven main sources of harm to patients:

1. medication errors
2. hospital-acquired infections for patients
3. hospital-acquired infections for staff (for instance, needlestick injuries)
4. falls
5. pressure ulcers
6. errors in the management of blood products
7. patient identification errors.

(Fedoruk 2012)

All of these errors fall within the scope of nursing practice. Nurses administer medications, manage infection control processes, monitor patients' mobility, check bedridden patients for pressure ulcers, and administer blood and blood products. The registered nurse is responsible for ensuring that organisational policies and procedures are followed where checking is required. Accuracy in patient identification, especially when administering blood, blood products or medications, is an important nursing function.

Such stringent checking procedures must be used when you are administering or checking other staff administering medications and blood or blood products to patients, or any procedures requiring accuracy in patient identification. In some instances you, as the registered nurse, will be signing off that patient identification was accurate. For example, when administering medications and blood or blood products, the following process may be used. The 'eight rights':

1. right time
2. right patient
3. right medication

WORKPLACE HEALTH AND SAFETY (WHS) – Nurses need to be aware of the policies and procedures relating to safe practice in their organisations, including the responsibilities of their employer, as well as their responsibilities as an employee under the Workplace Health and Safety (WHS) legislation in their state or territory.

4. right dose
5. right route
6. right effect
7. right documentation
8. right education.

The 'right' framework is used in most healthcare facilities, and you would probably have been introduced to a framework like this in your undergraduate program.

THEORY TO PRACTICE

You (as a new registered nurse) have arrived on duty for an afternoon shift in a busy surgical ward. The length of stay for patients in this unit is short but, because of hospital-acquired infections, two patients are staying longer. You are allocated your patients and, once you have received your handover and negotiated break times with the rest of the afternoon team, you go and introduce yourself to your patients. As you check the individual patient charts, you find that the two longer-term patients have been allocated to you (Mr Allan and Mr Carter). You check their charts, including their medication charts, and find that both patients are due for antibiotics to be administered intravenously over 1 hour in two hours' time. While you are talking with Mr Allan, he mentions that he is feeling uncomfortable in bed and asks if you could help make him comfortable. Mr Allan is rather large so you ask for help with moving him. On turning him, you notice his sacral area is very red and you ask whether he had been moved during the previous shift. Mr Allan says no—that the nurses in the morning were very busy and so he had not been helped out of bed and walked to the bathroom. He also tells you he has not had his anti-infection dose. Mr Carter, overhearing this, says he has not received his medications. You check both men's charts and find that all medications are charted as having been administered. You check their e-records and see written that both men had had a pleasant morning and had been mobilised for an hour. Yet the physical evidence (Mr Allan) would suggest otherwise.

Discussion Questions

1. What is the first thing you do? Do you report this as an incident to the team leader or ignore it?
2. Do you note this as an episode of 'missed care'?
3. Are these errors of omission or commission?
4. Do you see this as non-compliance with the NSQHSS and NMBA competency standards?
5. What steps would you take if the relatives of Mr Allan and Mr Carter complained about the poor quality of nursing care?

Violence in the Workplace

Unfortunately, violence in the healthcare workplace is increasing. Patients and their families can be violent, as can people affected by illicit substances and alcohol, and this is well documented in the media. All healthcare organisations will have policies and protocols that outline the management of violent members of the public, usually in emergency departments. A more insidious form of violence that is practiced in health care organisations is that of horizontal violence.

Horizontal/lateral violence

Horizontal or lateral violence refers to hostile and aggressive behaviour within a particular group of people (such as a team of healthcare workers). The phenomenon of horizontal or lateral violence is well documented in nursing literature and has been acknowledged as a 'critical global issue for healthcare organisations' (Hutchinson et al. 2010, p. E60). Bullying is a form of horizontal violence.

HORIZONTAL VIOLENCE – Antisocial behaviours between members of the same profession where one member(s) bullies another.

Non-physical violence in the healthcare workplace is often the result of bullying. 'Bullying' includes antisocial behaviours expressed as intimidation, verbal abuse, rudeness and threatening and embarrassing others. The effect of these antisocial behaviours on the staff member being bullied is psychological distress. If you are the target of bullying, this must be reported under the Work Health and Safety (WHS) legislation in your state or territory. Sustained bullying can cause severe psychological distress, which can manifest as physical and/or mental illness. All healthcare organisations, as part of their human resource management strategies, should give staff the opportunity to access employee assistance programs (EAPs) using external service providers.

Bullying in nursing appears to be becoming more prevalent (Hutchinson et al. 2010). New graduate nurses are particularly vulnerable to bullying and harassment in the workplace (Duchscher & Myrick 2008). Bullying is violence that has social and emotional elements. It manifests as antisocial and aggressive behaviour, which can escalate into physical violence, but usually bullies favour humiliating, denigrating, criticising and telling lies about the person or persons that are their targets. Bullies usually operate through weaving an intricate web of lies and denial. Because they are charming when doing this, it can take some time before this behaviour is recognised for what it truly is.

As a new registered nurse you are a prime candidate for bullying, especially if you are competent and knowledgeable—all the things the bullies probably are not. You will need to recognise bullying behaviours in order to defend yourself. Because these are covert, usually one-on-one between the bully and the victim, others may find it difficult to accept that bullying is occurring. Victims of bullying often develop physical and psychological symptoms that can result in ill health requiring medical treatment. Once this happens, you lose your confidence and self-esteem, and your work performance slips, which may be reflected in errors or poor decision-making. A good rule of thumb for recognising bullying behaviour when it is directed at you is: if you believe you are being bullied, you most probably are.

Strategies to deal with bullying and to stop being a victim include:

- Recognise the bullying behaviour for what it is—unacceptable behaviour from an inadequate person.
- Understand that it is not your fault—you are not responsible for the bully's behaviour.
- Understand that bullies are weak, vindictive people who can only feel good about themselves by diminishing others.
- Your hospital or agency will have human resource policies that deal with bullying—find out what these are and use them.
- Keep a written record of instances (date, time, context, nature) of bullying so that you have evidence when reporting.
- Be courageous and just refuse to play the bully's game—this can be difficult to do, but once it is, your confidence returns.

Report the bullying behaviour to senior management under the OHS&W legislation in your state.

- If you feel intimidated because the bully is your immediate manager, then you can go to the nurses union (in most states it will be the Australian Nursing & Midwifery Federation) for advice and support.
- In the most extreme cases you should seek legal advice.

It is important for you to recognise that bullying is unacceptable behaviour. You do not have to accept this sort of behaviour, and there are legislative and administrative processes in place to protect you. Remarks such as 'Don't worry, so and so always does this to new staff—it's part of your unofficial orientation' are wrong, inappropriate and only serve to support the bully.

Harassment in the Workplace

Closely aligned to bullying is harassment. Harassment, too, is becoming more prevalent. It may be based on gender, age, race or religion. Harassment can be as insidious as bullying, but the more overt forms are:

- sexual harrassment, such as inappropriate touching
- inappropriate comments
- 'jokey' emails that you might find offensive

- smutty jokes that others find offensive
- lies told about you
- being told off in front of others
- being insulted in front of others.

The more covert forms of harassment include:

- having your performance as a registered nurse continually criticised
- always being rostered onto the 'unsocial' shifts
- always being allocated the most difficult patients with little or no support
- being denied the opportunity to act in a more senior position, even though you have the competency and knowledge to do so
- being told that you are on probation and that your employment is contingent on favourable reports from other staff.

Just as bullying is unacceptable behaviour, so is harassment. The way to deal with harassment is by standing up for yourself. If you ask why you have been rostered on for the past five weekends or you have had a disproportionate number of late shifts compared to others then the person doing the rostering needs to be able to provide you with a rationale for this, a rationale that is focused on patient care and is not about others' social needs/wants.

Critical reflection

Reflect on your responses to unsociable behaviours from others. Are you able to stand up for yourself or do you give in to other people all the time? Role-play may be useful to identify unsociable behaviours as well as strategies to manage these situations.

- Have you ever felt unsafe at work? How did you manage the situation?
- What policies and support are available to you to deal with these situations?

Everyone's Responsibility

Bullying and harassment are not twenty-first-century phenomena, and we have all experienced bullying or harassment at some point in our lives. Which of the following situations can be described as harassment?

- having someone make inappropriate comments to you—comments that make you feel uncomfortable
- being questioned about your personal life in an open forum
- being criticised in front of others

- being rostered unfairly so that others can meet their social obligations
- being sent a smutty email.

There are elements of bullying and harassment in all of the above points.

Unfortunately, workplace violence is a fact of life for nurses and for all health professionals (Mercer 2007). We seem to live and work in an increasingly fast-paced society where violence is a by-product. Healthcare organisations have systems, policies and procedures to support safe practice. However, you too have a responsibility to ensure your own safety and the safety of the patients in your care. If you find yourself in a potentially dangerous situation, try and remove yourself from it. If you are unsure about carrying out a procedure, say so. Do not put yourself or your patients at risk.

SUMMARY

The core of nursing practice is the ability and capacity of individual nurses to be safe and competent practitioners. As a registered nurse, you will be expected to act within the bounds of legislation and the NMBA competencies. The organisation you work for will have policies and procedures that support safe systems of work and you must know what these are. Australia now has a national approach to managing safety and quality in healthcare organisations using the National Safety and Quality Health Service Standards developed by the Australian Commission on Safety and Quality in Health Care. These should be read and understood alongside the competency and registration standards for registered nurses from the Nursing and Midwifery Board of Australia.

Safe systems of work apply equally to direct care delivery to patients and to staff. Incidents occur because of system breakdowns such as workload stress or interruptions while carrying out nursing functions. When these incidents occur, you need to know how and to whom to report them so that they are managed effectively and so that strategies are implemented to minimise reoccurrences. As nurses, you should be able to identify missed episodes of nursing care and differentiate between errors of omission and commission in nursing practice and the how to deal with these.

Despite legislation, policies and procedures, antisocial behaviours such as bullying and harassment are prevalent in healthcare organisations. This chapter gives you some strategies to help you deal with these behaviours. The most important thing to remember is that you *do not have to put up with these behaviours*, which are reportable under WHS legislation.

The community expects safe, competent practitioners when they enter the healthcare system. Your responsibility is to ensure that these community expectations are met. Failure to do so can have negative consequences for you and for the patients in your care. Safe practice is an integral element of nursing in the twenty-first century.

Clinical governance, while relatively new, is linked to quality management that monitors safe practice. As a student nurse, you may not think that clinical governance is something you need to concern yourself with, but if you are delivering care to patients then you are engaging with the requirements of clinical governance.

Discussion questions

1. What do you understand safe nursing practice to be?

2. What are some sources of errors in the healthcare workplace?

3. How would you ensure safe nursing or midwifery practice?

4. How does clinical governance apply to you as a student nurse or midwife? How will it apply to you as a registered nurse or midwife?

5. What are some of the consequences of bullying in the workplace?

6. Do you think you will be able to recognise the signs of bullying?

Further Reading

Australian Commission on Safety and Quality in Health Care 2014, *National Safety and Quality Health Service Standards* (NSQHSS), Sydney, NSW.

Hutchinson, M, Vickers, M H, Jackson D & Wilkes L 2010, 'Bullying as circuits of power: an Australian Nursing Perspective', *Administrative Theory & Praxis*, vol. 32, no. 1, pp. 25–47.

Junhke, C, Mulbacher, AC 2013, 'Patient-centredness in integrated healthcare delivery systems—needs, expectations and priorities of organised healthcare systems', *International Journal of Integrated Care*, vol. 13m 28, pp 1–14.

Nursing and Midwifery Board of Australia 2013, *Competency Standards for the Registered Nurse*.

Nursing and Midwifery Board of Australia 2013, *Registration Standards for the Registered Nurse*.

SA Health Safety Learning System (SLS), *Incidents user guide*, available http://www.sahealth.sa.gov.au/wps/wcm/connect/010324804d4094b185aed7f08cd2a4a7/SLSIncidentsUserGuide-PHCS-SQ-20121029.pdf?MOD=AJPERES&CACHEID=010324804d4094b185aed7f08cd2a4a7

Sherwood, G 2011, 'Integrating quality and safety science in nursing education and practice', *Journal of Research in Nursing*, vol. 16, pp. 226–40 (http://jrn.sagepub.com/content.16/3/226).

Useful websites

Australian Commission on Quality and Safety in Health Care (ACSQHC): www.safetyandquality.gov.au

ACSQHC Clinical handover: www.safetyandquality.gov.au/internet/safety/publishing.nsf/content/PriorityProgram-05#Tools

ACSQHC Knowledge portal: www.safetyandquality.gov.au/internet/safety/publishing.nsf/content/inforx-lp

ACSQHC National inpatient medication chart: www.safetyandquality.gov.au/internet/safety/publishing.nsf/content/NIMC_001

ACSQHC patient identification advice: www.health.gov.au/internet/safety/publishing.nsf/Content/PriorityProgram-04

ACSQHC medication safety advice: www.safetyandquality.gov.au/internet/safety/publishing.nsf/Content/PriorityProgram-06

ACSQHC windows into safety and quality in healthcare: www.safetyandquality.gov.au/internet/safety/publishing.nsf/Content/windows-into-safety-and-quality-in-health-care-2008

Hand Hygiene Australia: www.hha.org.au

References

Ball, J, Murrells, T, Rafferty AM, Morrow, E & Griffiths, P 2014, ' "Care left undone" during nursing shifts: associations with workload and perceived quality of care', *BMJ Qual Saf* 23:116–25.

Balding, C & Maddock, A 2006, *South Australian safety and quality framework & strategy 2007–2011*, project report and supporting documents, Government of South Australia, Department of Health.

Duchscher, JEB & Myrick, F 2008, 'The prevailing winds of oppression: understanding the new graduate experience in acute care', *Nursing Forum*, vol. 43, no. 4, pp. 191–206.

Fedoruk, M 2014, 'Safety' in *Kozier & Erb's fundamentals of nursing*, 3rd Australasian edn, Pearson Publishing Australia, chapter 33.

Hand Hygiene Australia 2011, *The National hand hygiene initiative*, www.hha.org.au, accessed 11 October 2011.

Hutchinson, M, Jackson, D, Wilkes, L & Vickers, M 2010, 'A new model of bullying in the nursing workplace', *Advances in Nursing Science*, vol. 32, no. 2, pp. E60–71.

Kalisch, BJ, Landstrom G & Williams RA 2009, 'Missed nursing care: errors of omission', *Nursing Outlook*, 57 pp. 3–9.

Mercer, M 2007, 'The dark side of the job: violence in the emergency department', *Journal of Emergency Nursing*, vol. 33, pp. 257–61.

Sivitier, B 2008, *The newly qualified nurse's handbook*, Bailliere Tindall Elsevier, Edinburgh.

Wakefield, BJ 2014, 'Facing up to the reality of missed care', *BMJ Qual Saf* vol. 23, pp. 92–4.

12 Legal Responsibilities and Ethics

MARIA FEDORUK

LEARNING OBJECTIVES

By the end of this chapter you will be able to:

- differentiate between law and ethics
- discuss the relationship between law and ethics
- apply ethical principles to your practice
- analyse personal values that may influence your decision-making
- understand your role as a registered nurse in ethical healthcare issues.

KEY TERMS

Civil law
Common law
Consent to treatment
Contract of employment
Criminal law
Ethics
Registration
Statutory law

COMMON LAW –
Consists of cases decided by the courts using established common-law principles (Staunton & Chiarella 2013, p. 5).

STATUTORY LAW –
Consists of laws created by Parliament and embodied in documents known as Acts of Parliament, commonly referred to as 'legislation' (Staunton & Chiarella 2013, p. 5).

CRIMINAL LAW –
Rules of expected behaviours governing people's conduct in the community and backed by sanctions of punishment in relation to other people and their property (Staunton & Chiarella 2013, p. 8).

Introduction

This chapter provides an overview of the laws and ethics that underpin the practice of professional nursing in Australia. To understand your legal responsibilities as nurses it is important, as Staunton and Chiarella (2013 p. 1) point out, to have a 'rudimentary understanding of what the law is, where it comes from and how it operates'. As citizens of Australia or temporary residents, you are subject to the laws of Australia. Laws are enacted to protect the community and individuals from harm, and to protect personal property. There is also a judiciary process to manage transgressions. Staunton and Chiarella (2013) provide a historic overview of how the law, based on English law and principles, was developed in Australia, and how there are two main sources of law: **common law** and **statutory law** (p. 3).

The law is broadly categorised into two main areas: **criminal law** and **civil law**.

As student nurses, soon to be registered nurses, you are registered under the *National Law Act* (2012) which is regulated by the Nursing Midwifery Board of Australia (NMBA) working with the Australian Health Practitioner Regulation

Agency (AHPRA) to ensure all nurses are competent and fit to practice. The principal role of these regulatory agencies is to protect the public from harm. Registered nurses and midwives need to meet the **registration** standards that define the requirements that applicants, registrants or students need to meet in order to be registered. (NMBA 2012). The registration standards are available on the website of the NMBA (http://www.nursingmidwiferyboard.gov.au/Registration-Standards.aspx).

The NMBA also develops and endorses codes, guidelines and competency standard to guide the profession (http://www.nursingmidwiferyboard.gov.au/Codes-Guidelines-Statements/Codes-Guidelines.aspx). Included in this suite of codes, guidelines and standards are codes of ethics for nurses and midwives, and codes of professional conduct for nurses and midwives. These codes and guidelines specify the regulatory, behavioural and legal expectations of professional nurses and midwives. These standards, codes and guidelines are integral to your practice. You should always be aware of your legal responsibilities, because non-compliance with professional standards can cause you to lose your registration.

CIVIL LAW – Enables individuals, singly and collectively to resolve disputes and differences of a personal and property nature that arise between members of a community and which are unable to be resolved by the parties involved (Staunton & Chiarella, 2013, p. 9).

REGISTRATION – Occurs once a student nurse completes an accredited undergraduate program, meeting the registration standards requirements from the NMBA.

Critical reflection

Should nurses have to meet the requirements of the registration standards? Isn't having a degree enough of a qualification to become a registered nurse?

THEORY TO PRACTICE

You are on a clinical placement in an aged care facility. One day you observe one of the permanent staff (Jane) become impatient with a resident, forcing food and drink onto them. The resident becomes upset, coughs, splutters and spills food down the front of her nightgown. You go to help the registered nurse and the resident, but the registered nurse tells you to go away, the resident is just being difficult and it does not matter if she does not eat or drink, and, as she dirtied her clothes, she can stay in them. The nurse leaves to go to morning tea, telling you to do whatever you like with the resident. You stay with the resident, who finally settles down, and you ask if you can help her change her clothes. She tells you what clothes she would like and as you begin to undress her, you notice bruises on her arms. You ask about these but she is reluctant to discuss the bruises. Finally, she breaks down and tells you the registered nurse caused the bruises by grabbing her and pulling her when she was a little slow in moving. The resident had had a stroke several years ago and her mobility is slow. You discuss this with other nurses who just comment that it is just

Jane's way and not to worry about this, indicating this is a common occurrence and a number of residents are being hurt by Jane. But you do worry about this because it is a form of abuse.

Discussion Questions

1. Do you report this to the senior staff of the aged care facility?
2. Is this a reportable offence under the NMBA registration standards and the National Law (2012)?
3. If the senior management staff of the aged care facility do not address this issue, what are your responsibilities as a student nurse registered with AHPRA?
4. Would you not report this because you are afraid you will not receive a positive evaluation for your clinical placement?
5. Do the other nurses working in the aged care facility have responsibilities as defined by the registration standards and the National Law?

Nurses' Legal Responsibilities in Relation to Professional Practice

As beginning registered nurses, you will know by now the significance of understanding your legal responsibilities regarding your practice. You need to know your responsibilities under the *National Law Act 2012*, which regulates your entry into the nursing profession as a registered nurse, and is supported by the registration standards, and professional standards and codes of practice from the NMBA.

In the areas of clinical practice you should have an understanding of the legislation concerning **consent to treatment**, your contract of employment, report writing and the administration of drugs.

CONSENT TO TREATMENT – This is covered by an area of 'civil law relating to a trio of civil wrongs or torts concerned with 'trespass to the person' (Staunton & Chiarella 2013, p. 137).

Trespass to the person can include assault, battery and false imprisonment. Staunton and Chiarella continue their explanation of the importance of consent to treatment for nurses and other health professionals by describing it as 'defence to actions in assault, battery and false imprisonment. Consent, as you will have been taught, can be given verbally, in writing, or can be implied. (Staunton & Chiarella 2013, pp. 137–8). The elements of informed consent are:

- the consent is voluntarily and freely given
- that any consent given is properly informed
- That the person has the legal capacity to give it. (Staunton & Chiarella 2013, p. 144).

Critical reflection

Have you ever been present when the elements of informed consent were not present? Why did this happen and what were the consequences? In your tutorials, take the time to discuss the elements of informed consent and why these may be important.

As an employee of a healthcare organisation, you will be provided with a **contract of employment** detailing your conditions of employment and the employer's expectations. Contracts of employment are supported by legislation and you should have an awareness of the different pieces of legislation. It is important to have an understanding of *Work, Health & Safety Act 2012* because its focus is on workplace safety, including your personal safety.

Report writing is an essential component of nurses' work. The patient record should be an accurate and concise record of the patient's episode of healthcare. It is important to remember that there may be occasions when the patient record is used as evidence in court, but this is not the most important reason for keeping accurate health records. The records are also used for clinical teaching, and quality and safety audits. The following are some tips for maintaining accurate patient records, either paper based or electronic:

- You should never make an entry in the patient record on behalf of another nurse or health professional.
- Your reports should be accurate, concise and complete.
- Handwritten reports should be legible; illegible handwriting can lead to misinterpretation, which can result in hospital error.
- All reports should be objectively written. There should be no phrases like 'Mr M seemed to sleeping' or 'Mrs L appears to be shocked'. You need to provide specific clinical details.
- Entries in the patient record should be made as close as possible to an incident occurring. Critical incidents are reported as soon as possible, once the patient's condition is stabilised. Each state and territory Department of Health has its own incident reporting system and you should be aware of this.
- You should not use abbreviations unless they are specific to a healthcare organisation.
- Make sure you know the exact meaning of any medical terminology you are going to use.
- Any errors made while making an entry in the patient record should have a line drawn through them and be initialled. Never obliterate an incorrect entry.

CONTRACT OF EMPLOYMENT – The basis of a health professional's relationship with an employer is that of contract where the employer has the power to direct the manner in which an employee performs work (McIllwraith & Madden 2014, p. 349).

MARIA FEDORUK

There are some general guiding principles for managing clinical and patient documentation:

- The patient record should be comprehensive and complete.
- The patient record should be patient centred and collaborative.
- The patient record should be confidential.

(Staunton & Chiarella 2013)

The administration of drugs, medication administration is another nursing function. In your undergraduate program, you will have been shown how to administer medications safely and correctly, yet there is still a high incidence of medication errors occurring in health and aged care facilities nationally. The figures for hospital admissions are 5.6 per cent in the general population, 30.4 per cent of admissions in the elderly to 3.3 per cent of paediatric admissions. As registered nurses and enrolled nurses endorsed to administer medications, you have a responsibility to know the regulations covering medication administration (Staunton & Chiarella 2013, p. 211).

Ethics

ETHICS – Refers to the various ways of thinking and understanding how to live a moral life.

Johnstone (2009) explains that **ethics** is a broad generic term, used to refer to the various ways of thinking and understanding how to live a moral life. Kerridge et al. in Staunton and Chiarella (2013 p. 27) describe 'ethics' as prescriptive—concerned with what we should do rather than what we actually do. Johnstone (2009) describes' bioethics' as the systematic study of the moral dimensions of health and life sciences, using different ethical methodologies. You will be aware of such bioethical issues as organ donation, reproductive technology issues, cosmetic surgery for adolescents and any issues where peoples' belief and values systems are challenged because from time to time they attract media attention, and you will have to draw your own conclusions, based on your own values and belief systems. 'Nursing ethics' can be defined broadly as the exploration of all kinds of ethical and bioethical issues from a nursing theory and practice perspective (Johnstone 2009).

Staunton and Chiarella (2013 p. 37) provide an ethical decision framework which you might want to use in your study groups to work through a case study. The framework has the following elements:

- State the problem clearly—consider the problem within its context and distinguish between ethical and other issues such as medical and sociocultural. Examine the meanings of value-laden terms such as 'quality of life'.
- Get the facts—take the time to get as many facts about the problem as possible before trying to arrive at a solution.

- Consider the fundamental principles—apply each one to the dilemma.
- Look at the problem from a different perspective.
- Identify any ethical conflicts.
- Consider the law—any legal concepts or laws, and how these might guide decision-making; examine the relationship between the ethical–clinical decision and the law.
- Make an ethical decision and justify it.

However, ethics is not law, empirical data, policies, codes or guidelines, religion or morality, or following the orders of a manager (Staunton & Chiarella 2013, p. 28). There are four major ethical principles:

- *Autonomy*—the right to self-determination and, from a patient perspective, the right of individuals to make choices about treatment without interference from external parties, including healthcare teams, even when those choices differ from that of health professionals.
- *Non-maleficence*—the principle of doing no harm. Nurses have a professional responsibility to avoid harming patients and to practice competently.
- *Beneficence*—the principle of doing good or acting for the benefit of others. All nursing practice is directed at achieving positive benefits for others.
- *Justice*—this has two meanings in the field of ethics: 'fairness', and the equal distribution of burdens and benefits. This principle is about treating all patients fairly, especially in relation to access to scarce resources in the healthcare system (Staunton and Chiarella 2013, pp. 34–5).

THEORY TO PRACTICE

A tragic outcome

Mr B, an 80-year-old man, is admitted to a clinical unit with chronic hypertension and mild left ventricular failure. He is admitted for elective surgery—trans-urethral resection of the prostate. He is accompanied by his 74-year-old sister, Ms W, who informs the nursing staff that they live together in the country, approximately 250 kilometres away from the hospital. To get to the hospital, they had to catch a bus at 7 am in their town. They have no living relatives or close friends they can call on for help following Mr B's discharge from hospital.

While completing Mr B's assessment, both brother and sister tell the nursing staff that they enjoy good health apart from the usual 'getting old' things. Both say they are active when at home and enjoy gardening and bowls at their local club.

Mr B has his surgery on a Tuesday and is discharged on the following Saturday, with an indwelling catheter. Prior to discharge, his sister is shown how to manage the catheter, how to change the catheter bag and how to attach the night-time bag.

Ms W does not want to appear to be 'difficult' so she does not ask the nurse any questions about care of the catheter.

They travel home on the bus, and when they arrive home Mr B remembers he gave his antihypertensive tablets to a nurse on admission and forgot to get them back. His sister rings the hospital and the ward and explains the situation, but is told by the registered nurse that she cannot do anything about it because the drugs have been returned to the pharmacy, as per hospital policy, and the pharmacy is now closed. Because they have returned to the country, there is no way she can get the medication to them. Ms W begins to get upset and panic, but the registered nurse assures her that the community nursing service have been advised of Mr B's discharge and will contact them later in the evening.

Ms W contacts the community nursing service and is told someone will be there shortly once they find the faxed referral. After this, Ms W notices that her brother seems drowsy, his movements are slow and his speech is slurred. She contacts the community nursing service again, explaining her brother's clinical condition. The nurse explains that there is no referral from the hospital, but tells her a nurse will come within thirty minutes.

However, the community nurses are particularly busy and it is more than an hour before a registered nurse arrives. During this time, Ms W tries to rouse her brother but he seems to be increasingly drowsy. Thinking that there might be some antihypertensive tablets in the medication cupboard, Ms W climbs onto a chair to look for them. The chair wobbles, and Ms W falls and fractures the neck of her right femur. When the community nurse arrives at their home, she finds Ms W on the floor in pain and Mr B unconscious in his chair.

The community nurse rings for an ambulance to take brother and sister to the local hospital for initial treatment, but Mr B passes away in the ambulance. He had had a cerebrovascular accident and the case is referred to the coroner. Ms W has a total hip replacement, but is not told of her brother's death for at least two days following her surgery.

Discussion Questions

1. Referring to the ethical principles above, discuss the questions listed below.
2. Identify the ethical principles in this case study.
3. If you were the hospital nurse, would you have done anything differently?
4. Would you have told Ms W her brother had passed away sooner?
5. Were there any legal issues in this case study?
6. Which ethical principle is the most important in this case?

Two other ethical principles which you may wish to consider are:

- *Fidelity*—the duty to be faithful to commitments and involves maintaining confidentiality, privacy and trust. To whom did the nurse owe fidelity in the case study above—the patient, the patient's family or the hospital?
- *Veracity*—the duty to tell the truth. Two situations in which this principle may become an issue are:
  - when a patient asks for their diagnosis and the medical staff have not yet discussed it with them
  - when you witness a critical incident (such as a medication error) by a colleague which results in a negative outcome for a patient and you are asked by the nurse manager to give an accurate report of the incident. Do you tell the truth?

Patient Rights

In Australia, in 2009 the Council of Australian Governments (COAG) released the *Australian Charter of Healthcare Rights*.

The charter is underpinned by three principles:

- Everyone has the right to be able to access healthcare and this right is essential for the Charter to be meaningful.
- The Australian Government commits to international agreements about human rights which recognise everyone's right to have the highest possible standard of physical and mental health.
- Australia is a society made up of people from different cultures and ways of life and the Charter recognises and respects these differences.

(ACSQH 2010, p. 1)

Under the charter, all citizens have:

- a right to access healthcare
- a right to receive safe and high-quality care
- a right to be shown respect, dignity and consideration
- a right to be informed about services, treatment options and costs in a clear and open way
- a right to be included in decisions and choices about their care
- a right to privacy and confidentiality of their personal information
- a right to comment on their care and to have their concerns addressed.

(adapted from ACSQH 2010)

Mental health

There is a legislative approach to treating health (think back to the section on informed consent), with each state and territory having similar approaches based on the following areas:

- defining what persons come within the legislation
- the process which must be followed to admit, detain and treat persons under the legislation
- provision for what types of treatment may be given under the legislation and the processes to be followed to do so
- the recognition of the fundamental rights of persons admitted, detained and treated under the legislation
- provision of appropriate review and appeal mechanisms to ensure that persons are not inappropriately detained and that while they are detained their civil rights are protected

(Staunton & Chiarella 2013, p. 321)

The framework for ensuring that people with a mental health illness receive the most appropriate treatment without loss of dignity or civil liberties is enshrined in legislation. All states and territories have legislation that is consistent with the United Nation's *Principles with Mental Health Care*. These principles also protect the individual from any form of exploitation, any form of discrimination, and maintain their cultural, civic, political, social and civic rights.

Advance directives

Advance directives or 'living wills' are a recent phenomenon. They ensure that patient rights are honoured when the patient no longer has the capacity to refuse treatment. In Australia, some states and territories have legislated for advance directives: South Australia has the *Consent to Treatment and Palliative Care Act 1995*; Victoria has the *Medical Treatment Act 1988*, the *Medical Treatment (Enduring Power of Attorney) Act 1990* and the *Medical Treatment (Agents) Act 1992* and the Northern Territory has the *Natural Death Act 1988*.

It is also worth noting that, in Australia, you may come across patients who have given their relatives an 'enduring medical power of attorney', which grants relatives the legal right to make decisions on behalf of the patient in all medical matters.

At some point you may be asked to witness legal documents for patients—it is advisable to be cautious, and not do this. While, as an adult, you are legally entitled to be a witness, it is not advisable to do so as an employee. Your healthcare organisation will have administrative staff with the designated responsibility to do this.

Non-Clinical Ethical Issues

The preceding section considered ethical principles from a clinical perspective but, as a registered nurse, you will be faced with ethical dilemmas that for the purposes of this section may be considered non-clinical or administrative. Some examples include instances of:

- perceived unsafe staffing levels in terms of skill levels and knowledge, rather than numbers of staff
- poor nursing practice
- unprofessional behaviours from other nurses or other health professionals
- covering up of nurse-initiated mistakes or errors
- errors or poor practice from other health professionals.

As a registered nurse, what would you do if you observed another health professional engaging in unsafe practices? Would you:

- report this using the organisational processes for reporting these sorts of incidents?
- speak to the other health professional outlining your concerns?
- do nothing?

Critical reflection

Think back to your student nurse days, when you were on clinical placement. Did you observe other nurses 'cutting corners' in order to finish their work on time—not having medications checked when they should? Does this fall under the banner of ethical misconduct? Which ethical principle is breached? Now, fast-forward to the present, and you are the registered nurse—do you believe it is alright to cut corners when you are on a busy shift because usually nothing bad happens—patients really don't know anything and they are Okay. Or, if you do question unsafe practices, the response is 'Oh we always do it this way, nothing bad ever happens.' Another reason for cutting corners: 'if we do not finish our work on time we get into trouble'. From what you now know, are any of these reasons justifiable?

Whistleblowing

Whistleblowing in the healthcare sector is achieving prominence in the media, with cases of unsafe and incompetent practices by health professionals being reported. Your registration as a registered nurse is dependent on you being able to show evidence of safe, competent and ethical practice (your professional portfolio) to the national registering authority, the Australian Health Practitioner Regulation

Agency. These professional portfolios will be subject to random audits in the coming years, as a quality management strategy. Inherent in your legal and ethical responsibility to be a safe, competent nurse is your duty to report areas of unsafe, incompetent practice from other health professionals, including nurse colleagues.

Whistleblowing is not specific to healthcare. In the corporate world, whistleblowing usually occurs around financial fraud, and it can result in companies collapsing and managers being jailed.

In healthcare, apart from whistleblowing about unsafe practices, there have also been cases of faulty medical devices and drugs having negative outcomes for patients. These are usually reported in the media in the context of litigation, with victims seeking legal reparation for pain and suffering.

It should be noted that whistleblowing does not always result in sensationalised media attention; it can be managed appropriately and sensitively by organisations and regulatory agencies.

Nurse whistleblowers have been defined as nurses 'who identify incompetent, unethical or illegal situations in the workplace and report it to someone who has the power to stop the wrong' (McDonald & Ahern in Firtko & Jackson 2005, p. 52). A more generic definition of whistleblowing, provided by Firtko and Jackson (2005, p. 52), is 'the reporting of information to an individual, group or body that is not part of an organisation's usual problem-solving strategy'. As a registered nurse, you have a duty of care not to harm patients, either directly or indirectly. All healthcare organisations in Australia are mandated to provide safe and competent health services. This is reflected in standards, clinical protocols, policies and procedures, and you are expected to work within these frameworks. However, reporting others for wrongdoing poses ethical dilemmas for nurses, and you have to make a decision in relation to your values, belief systems and regulatory obligations.

Deciding whether to be a whistleblower presents you with an ethical dilemma that challenges your core personal and professional values. It may make you question the level of the responsibilities you have to patients, the community, your profession and your employer (Firtko & Jackson 2005). These are all issues you will have to grapple with in coming to a decision on the best way to act in the circumstances. There may be risks to you in reporting incidents. You may be labelled as a troublemaker and this may have an impact on your future employment prospects. In extreme cases, this may result in your being dismissed from the organisation. There may also be risks to the organisation from legal actions taken by patients and/or their relatives. Another thing to remember is that whistleblowing does not often result in an immediate positive outcome, especially if legal proceedings are initiated. It is important to be aware of the risks of whistleblowing. This is not intended to discourage or scare you, but, instead, to remind you of your professional responsibilities to ensure safe practice and ensure patients and other staff members come to no harm.

Therefore, before proceeding down the whistleblower path you should:

- use all the processes available in the organisation to report potential incidents that can cause harm to staff or patients
- discuss your concerns with a mentor or someone who may be able to intervene to stop the poor behaviour
- collect evidence relating to the incidents and be very certain of your facts. You will need objectivity not subjectivity when collating your evidence.
- be very sure of organisational policies and procedures, and the laws governing practice
- seek advice from an external party such as an industrial organisation or even a lawyer.

Most states and territories have legislation to protect whistleblowers. For example in South Australia there is the *Whistleblowers Protection Act 1993*. It is wise to check your legal status under the relevant legislation if you find yourself in a whistleblowing situation.

SUMMARY

This chapter has provided an overview of the legal responsibilities of the registered nurse when providing care to patients. The chapter covers the requirements for registration under the National Law and the NMBA registration standards. It points out the relevant pieces of legislation that underpin core nursing functions and employment. There is also a section on professional regulation of the nursing profession.

These core nursing functions include report writing, medication administration and consent to treatment.

The chapter also discusses the differences between law and ethics, and define nursing ethics and bioethics. There is an ethical decision-making framework which you might find useful in working through a clinical issue or problem that has both ethical and legal dimensions.

Discussion questions

1. Have you given any consideration to how you might manage unethical behaviours in the workplace?

2. Have you witnessed any unethical behaviour in the workplace? How was it managed? Was it reported? How were the individuals involved in these matters managed?

3. Why is it important for nurses and for all health professionals to comply with ethical codes of conduct?

MARIA FEDORUK

Further Reading

Johnstone MJ 2009, *Bioethics: a nursing perspective*, 5th edn, Churchill Livingstone, Elsevier NSW.

MacIlwraith, J & Madden, B 2010, *Health care and the law*, 5th edn, Thomson Reuters (Professional) Australia Limited, Sydney.

Staunton, P & Chiarella, M 2013, *Law for nurses and midwives*, 7th edn, Churchill Livingstone, Elsevier NSW.

Useful websites

Australian Health Practitioner Regulation Agency, legislation: www.ahpra.gov.au/ Legislation-and-Publications/Legislation.aspx

Nurses and Midwifery Board of Australia www.nmba.gov.au

References

Australian Commission on Safety and Quality in Health Care 2010, *Australian charter of healthcare rights*, Australian Government, Canberra, www.safetyandquality.gov.au/ internet/safety/publishing.nsf/Content/com-pubs_ACHR-pdf-01-con/$File/17537-charter.pdf accessed 17/4/14.

Australian Government, Department of Employment 2012, *Work, Health and Safety Act 2012*.

Firtko, A & Jackson, D 2005, 'Do the ends justify the means? Nursing and the dilemma of whistleblowing,' *Australian Journal of Advanced Nursing*, vol. 23, no. 1, pp. 51–6.

International Council of Nurses 2006, *The ICN code of ethics for nurses*, International Council of Nurses, Geneva, www.icn.ch/images/stories/documents/about/icncode_english.pdf accessed 17/4/14.

McIlwraith, J & Madden, B 2014, *Health care and the law*, 6th edn, Thomson Reuters (Professional) Australia, Ltd, NSW, Lawbook Co.

Staunton, P & Chiarella, M 2013 *Law for nurses and midwives*, 7th edn, Churchill Livingstone Elsevier Australia, NSW.

Health Information Systems and Technologies

13

MARIA FEDORUK

LEARNING OBJECTIVES

After reading this chapter, you will be able to:

- explain the significance of data management for decision-making in nursing practice
- define and describe computer applications used in clinical nursing practice in your healthcare environment
- critically analyse the effectiveness of nursing information systems to safe, competent nursing care
- analyse information needs required for your nursing practice
- use nursing information systems and technologies to integrate research-based evidence into nursing practice.

KEY TERMS

Competencies
eHealth
mHealth
Nursing informatics

Introduction

This chapter provides you with a brief overview of how information and communication technologies are being introduced into healthcare organisations across the country, to manage and disseminate clinical corporate information and to inform decision-making. To understand the new nursing specialisation of nursing informatics, it is important to understand how information and communication technologies are transforming nurses' work spaces and how this is adding the competency of 'knowledge worker' to the role and function of the nurse. These technologies are providing nurses with real-time clinical information which has to be translated, where appropriate, into nursing actions.

Nurses as frontline workers in healthcare organisations are 'knowledge workers', using competencies such as 'analysis, synthesis and cross-disciplinary coordination' (Zang et al. 2012, p. 1621). As knowledge workers, nurses principally interact with patient health information by means of the electronic health record. Nurses provide and collect information to plan and coordinate patient care.

eHEALTH – the combined use of communication and information technology in the healthcare sector to deliver the right information to the right person at the right time in a secure electronic environment, to ensure the optimal delivery of safe, quality care to patients. eHealth is the infrastructure that supports information exchange between all healthcare professionals and patients.

In 2008, Australian Health Ministers, through the Australian Health Ministers' Advisory Council (AHMAC), commissioned a private consulting firm to develop a strategic and coordinated national approach to the implementation of **eHealth**. One of the outcomes of the national ehealth strategy has been the implementation of the new electronic patient record (Department of Health 2012).

Australia's healthcare system is a large and complex industry that employs close to 1 million people, and provides health services to approximately 22 million people located in diverse geographical and socio-economic areas in all states and territories. The dissemination of accurate and timely information is essential for the provision of safe, quality care to patients who may be in hospitals or receiving health services in the community. It is important to note that health services are delivered by multidisciplinary health teams who use information and communication technologies to communicate patient information. Figure 13.1 shows a diagrammatic representation of information flows in a healthcare system. You can see the number of health practitioners that may be involved in the process.

FIGURE 13.1 DIAGRAMMATIC REPRESENTATION OF INFORMATION FLOWS IN A HEALTHCARE SYSTEM

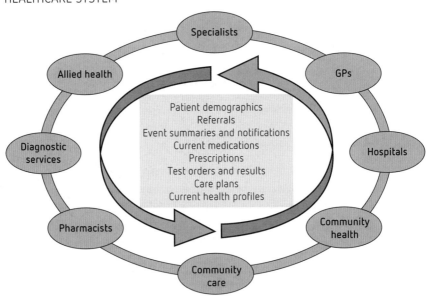

Source: National E-Health Strategy. Australian Health Ministers' Conference (2008). Victorian Department of Human Services on behalf of the Australian Health Ministers' Conference http://www.ehealth.gov.au/internet/ehealth/publishing.nsf/content/home.

Up until 2012, the health information environment was fragmented, with information held in various locations by various people, and was paper based;

all of which created barriers to the effective sharing of information, made more difficult because of Australia's multiple health services boundaries and geographical distances (AHMAC 2008, p. 3). This essentially manual system of sharing information increased the potential for error and inefficiency. This is apparent when you consider the numbers of point-of-service interactions between multiple service providers and patients. Nurses are an integral component of this information-sharing process and therefore need to develop the competencies for managing patient information to support their clinical decision-making, and care planning with a multidisciplinary team. In figure 13.1, nurses work in and with all the components listed.

eHealth

The Australian healthcare system is one of the best in the world, providing universal access to all Australian citizens to a quality healthcare system, and the community expects this to continue (AHMC 2008). But an ageing population and increases in chronic disease, demands for services and the costs associated with providing health services require changes to how health services are delivered and managed. Hence, the national eHealth strategy was implemented to increase efficiencies, reduce hospital errors, and improve the safety and quality of health services delivered. Therefore, eHealth is intended to address multiple issues in the healthcare system.

As beginning registered nurses, it is important for you to understand how the healthcare system is being reformed through the use of information and communication technologies. These technologies will change how nurses work and interact with patients and other healthcare professionals, and nurses need to develop information literacy competencies to underpin emerging nursing informatics competencies. This is occurring at the same time as health consumer literacy is increasing, because the health consumer has the capacity to access health-related information electronically.

The healthcare and nursing literature reports favourably on the use of eHealth technologies, but it is always important to take notice of the not-so-positive reports. For example, Ash et al. (2004), reporting the results of three separate studies conducted in the United States, the Netherlands and Australia, using the same methodologies, found that there were unintended consequences, 'patient care information related system errors' (p. 104). These unintended system errors included errors in the process of entering and retrieving information. Because healthcare environments are complex and dynamic, and staff are often time-poor, the potential for entering and retrieving information errors is high. A second source of system error related to communication and coordination of information. Ash et al. (2004, p. 105) comment that 'computers can undermine communication about and coordination of events and activities' through misrepresenting healthcare work and interactions as linear and predictable, and 'misrepresenting communication as information transfer'. But, as you know, in a real-world situation these interactions are rarely linear, nor is all communication between health professionals information transfer.

Other writers discuss the barriers to the effective use of eHealth technologies, including a lack of awareness and a lack confidence in using these technologies among healthcare consumers and health professionals, with concerns expressed about privacy and security relating to health information (Fairbrother et al. 2014; Harris et al. 2012).

These new technologies are central to your practice as a registered nurse now and into the future; they are becoming an integral part of your work, are evident in your nursing practice standards and will be included in your employment documentation, such as your employment contract, and person and job specification.

Critical reflection

You may wish to consider how you are going to develop as a knowledge worker in healthcare, thus ensuring continued employability as a registered nurse into the future.

While on clinical placements, you will have noticed the use of information and communication technologies in hospitals and other healthcare agencies. Departments of Health in Australian states and territories will have implemented information and communication technologies in the public healthcare agencies to comply with the national eHealth strategy. You should access the websites for the Department of Health in your state or territory to find out what is happening in your healthcare system. For example, the Department of Health in South Australia is rolling out the Enterprise Patient Administration System (EPAS) across the public healthcare system (http://www.sahealth.sa.gov.au/wps/wcm/connect/ Public+Content/SA+Health+Internet/Search/Search+results).

Nurses, as the largest employee group in healthcare organisations, play a pivotal role in managing patient information. Nurses, therefore, have to develop competencies in nursing informatics if they are to take and maintain the lead role in patient care delivery.

Nursing Informatics

Nursing informatics is a subset of health informatics, the science that uses health and population data to plan health services into the future, identify disease and treatment trends, and global workforce requirements. At the healthcare organisational level, health informatics data report on clinical practices and patient activity, measure organisational performance, and supports the development of a safety and quality environment. Nursing informatics provides the nurse-generated information for health informatics (Moren et al. 2013).

Nurses work in all healthcare environments and are becoming more dependent on electronic information (Hovenga 2013, p. 14).

Nurses working in the twenty-first century need to develop higher-order critical thinking competencies to be able to analyse the information they will be working with, in order to make clinical decisions and to plan safe, quality patient care. Strachan et al. (2011, p. 1) notes that nursing informatics not only supports nurses in delivering care to patients but also emphasises 'patient centredness, nursing effectiveness and patient safety'. Nursing informatics, as a part of information technology initiatives in healthcare organisations, have the potential to change nurses' work and communication. Already, you will have become aware of this through your lectures and clinical placements. Nursing informatics and information literacy **competencies** are interdependent, and this is why your nursing studies focus on critical thinking, analysis and information management.

Nurses, as members of the health workforce most intimately involved in delivering patient care, will possess large amounts of information about patients in their care. This information is personal and contains clinical information specific to a patient that is confidential. In the past, nurses managed this information manually, it was paper-based and usually not kept in one place. At times, nurses forgot to communicate relevant information to other health professionals, resulting in poor outcomes for patients. The use of web-based technologies to manage clinical information is improving nursing care and resulting in better outcomes for patients.

At the end of this chapter there are a number of web links to nursing informatics associations—national and international. These provide information that will help you develop your nursing informatics competencies.

Nursing Informatics Competencies

Chang et al (2011) report on a research study in Taiwan that focused on the nursing informatics competencies required of nurses working in Taiwan. The study provided a list of nursing informatics required of nurses working in the United

NURSING INFORMATICS – science and practice integrates nursing, its information and knowledge and their management with information and communication technologies to promote the health of people, families and communities worldwide (Hovenga 2013, p. 14).

COMPETENCIES – Capabilities or abilities that include both intent and action that link directly to how well a person performs completing tasks.

States and Taiwan. This study publishes nursing informatics competencies for beginning registered nurses and for experienced nurses.

Examples of nursing informatics competencies

Beginning registered nurses

The beginning registered nurse is able to:

- use decision support systems for clinical decision-making
- use information search tools
- locate evidence to support and problem-solve clinical practice issues
- analyse patient information needs and access resources to address identified needs
- apply the principles of data integrity and professional ethics, and adhere to the legal requirements for patient confidentiality and data security
- use information to ensure safety and quality in nursing care delivery.

Experienced registered nurses

The experienced registered nurse is able to:

- synthesise data from more than one source and apply to practice
- use information and communication technologies to manage care delivery, empower patients and enhance decision-making
- critically analyse data, information and knowledge for specific evidence-based practice situations
- assess the quality, accuracy, reliability and validity of health information available on the internet
- use patient data in safety and quality programs
- synthesise best practice evidence and translate this into nursing practice
- integrate technologies into clinical practice through patient education
- convert information needs to answerable questions.

(adapted from Chang et al. 2011, p. 335)

As you can see from the nursing informatics competencies presented above, the development of these competencies takes time, and you should use these examples to begin developing your own nursing informatics competencies. These competencies focus on all areas of nursing practice.

For nurses and other clinicians, the benefits of information technologies and the data that can be accessed include:

- access to clinical information at the point of care
- the use of a single clinical record supports improved communication and collaboration among health professionals

- there is more time to deliver care to patients
- less time is spent in creating paper-based documentation
- creation of an auditable record of care delivered to patients
- there is real-time integration of mobile device vital sign information directly into the patient's record
- data for measuring quality and patient care outcomes
- alerts that advance patient safety
- the use of standardise language to document care.

(Simpson 2011, p. 1)

While nurses worldwide are accepting the use of technology in providing care to patients, there are ethical dimensions to be considered. These centre primarily around confidentiality and privacy relating to patient information, as well as access to this information. Technically, as a staff member of a healthcare organisation, you will have a security code to access the patient information in that organisation, as well as other information specific and confidential to the organisation. This is something to be aware of, because breaches of this trust can result in instant dismissal from the organisation.

Critical reflection

Reflect on the data or information you have collected while caring for patients. How did you manage this information? How did it influence your care planning and delivery to patients?

While nursing informatics is a relatively new domain of nursing practice, information and communication technologies will continue to develop and evolve, as will you if you are to deliver safe, competent nursing care and become a valued member of a multidisciplinary team.

THEORY TO PRACTICE

You are a student nurse on your final clinical placement in an orthopaedic ward in a metropolitan tertiary hospital. During your placement period, a number of elderly patients (usually admitted from aged care facilities for different procedures), developed pressure ulcers; at least two patients had infected ulcers, even though the care plans indicated that pressure ulcer management had been factored into the care plan. The high incidence of pressure ulcers is concerning because patients are having to spend a longer time in hospital, which is distressing to them. Their families are also upset and have complained to senior management about the poor quality of care being delivered. Senior management asks why this is occurring and what is being done to address these issues. All the elderly patients are at risk of developing infections. A multidisciplinary team meeting is called to discuss the issues and, as a member of the team, you attend as well.

The Clinical Nurse Specialist (CNS) presents the clinical data, and a discussion occurs about different treatment options, including prophylactic antibiotic therapy for the non-infected patients. The CNS asks you if you would like to be involved in the problem-solving exercise by finding research-based evidence that would help resolve these particular issues. You agree to do this because you still have several weeks of the placement to complete. You see it as an interesting project and you can include your participation in this quality improvement activity in your e-portfolio.

While caring for patients, you happen to mention this little project, and one of the patients tells you they have Googled pressure ulcers and they ask you to look at the information they have and to tell them if it would be safe to put honey on their ulcer because honey, according to their information, will help heal the ulcer.

Discussion Questions

1. How would you manage the patient's information and their questions?
2. How would you begin your information search? What would you do first?
3. What data bases will you access? Will you begin with Google? Wikipedia?
4. Will you ask for help to analyse the information you retrieve?
5. What sort of data and information will you retrieve?
6. How will you present your information to the multidisciplinary team?

---

mHealth

mHEALTH —
Healthcare services that are or accessed by mobile devices such as mobile phones, smartphones, laptops and tablets to collect, retrieve and/or deliver health information.

mHealth is the use of mobile devices (e.g. smart phones, laptops, tablets and iPads) to collect, retrieve and deliver health information (Boisvert, 2012, p. 44). mHealth differs from eHealth and telemedicine because it is 'a subset of services delivered provided and accessed through mobile devices any place any time', as long there is wireless internet or cellular access (p. 44). The World Health Organization (2011) estimates that there are 5 billion mobile phone subscriptions in the world, with over 85% of the world's population covered by commercial wireless signal (p. 5). These networks are becoming increasingly sophisticated, with faster speeds of data transmission making it easier to access, deliver and manage data.

In developing countries, mobile technologies are used to communicate with people in remote communities, as well as providing disease-prevention strategies or notifying of disease outbreaks (WHO 2011).

An example of how mobile technologies are used in health is provided by health call centres and counselling centres. In some organisations, health call centres are used to triage patients who are potentially at risk. At a more basic level, how many of you now have your dental or GP appointments confirmed by SMS? Bauer et al. (2014) discusses the use of mobile health apps to support patients in managing their own healthcare and developing their own health literacy. However, the increasing sophistication of mobile technologies provides opportunities to introduce them into more mainstream healthcare.

Lederman et al. (2014) bring a cautionary note to the credibility of materials downloaded from the numerous sites now available to everyone. A question for you—how would you assess the credibility of information presented from an online forum by an anonymous donor? This is one of the risks associated with the widespread use of internet material. Similarly, in the healthcare workplace, what strategies are in place to monitor the credibility of clinical information being communicated to you?

Social media

The improved functionality of mobile devices has increased the attractiveness of social media as a communication tool for higher education studies (Usher et al. 2014). Their research has shown that, for first-year and final-year students in the health disciplines, online media is the preferred source of information and that students engage with social media platforms. However, there needs to be a word of caution here, around misuses of social media relating to academic performance and, where students go out on clinical placement, breaches of confidentiality and privacy of healthcare consumers and of the healthcare facility. There is widespread use of social media platforms in workplaces—indeed, some places encourage this form of communication—but there needs to be an awareness of professional boundaries while at work. Griffiths et al. (2012) consider a future where social networks are central to the delivery of healthcare. This is a consequence of the extensive global social networking 'mediated by information and communication' which is changing the way the world operates (p.2233). Consider how socially networked you are now, and what your principal forms of communication are— now translate this to the workplace. Do you see any differences between how society operated in the past and today? So, social networking and media are changing how we work and live in the world.

Lindley and Fernando (2013, p. 5) discuss the many issues, positive and negative, related to the rapid proliferation of mHealth technologies in clinical settings, often without guidelines for best practice use; the significant implications for clinical care, professional practice and the education of health professionals.

MARIA FEDORUK

They advise that while there are benefits, there are also significant risks around quality and safety issues for clinical care. The potential benefits include resource maximisation such as storing data on one device, convenience, speedier access to information, ease of use and use in work practices. (Kabashiki, 2013) provides positive commentary about how eHealth technologies will continue to improve health services because the healthcare consumer becomes a partner in their own healthcare.

Another technology which is gaining currency in healthcare is that of virtual communities, where users practice in online communities. Some of you may have already been introduced to virtual communities in your studies, with many universities adapting this technology into a teaching tool and resource. The following is a link to a YouTube presentation from the National eHealth Transition Authority: http://www.youtube.com/watch?v=JwDTxvkBk-I.

SUMMARY

This chapter looked at how information and communication technologies have changed workplace behaviours, and the practices of health professionals, including nurses. Nurses are now knowledge workers, with information literacy competencies underpinning their nurse informatics competencies.

Electronic and communication technologies, and the increased use of mobile technologies, are changing the healthcare landscape and the way in which nurses work. These technologies provide nurses with opportunities to assume leadership roles, especially in developing new and innovative ways of delivering care to patients. This can include moving care into cyberspace and patients into virtual nursing and healthcare practices. Social networks such as Facebook, Twitter and YouTube all have the potential to change the nurse–patient interaction, and the relationships between all health professionals.

Discussion questions

1. In your time as a student nurse, how have you noticed a change in the technologies being used in healthcare organisations?

2. Has there been a change in your professional interactions because of these technologies?

3. How comfortable are you working with these technologies?

4. How confident are you in retrieving clinical information, analysing it and then making a patient care decision?

5. Do you see yourself as a knowledge worker?

6. What are the advantages of using eHealth and mHealth technologies in nursing practice?

Further Reading

Ball, MJ, Douglas, JV & Walker PH (eds) 2011, *Nursing informatics*, Springer, London.

World Health Organization 2011, *mHealth. New horizons for health through mobile technologies*, Global Observatory, for e Health series, Volume 3.

Useful websites

Australian College of Nursing 2013—Nurse Click http://www.acn.edu.au/sites/default/files/publications/nurseclick/acn_nurseclick_august_2013_non-member.pdf. This link takes you to an article on nursing informatics by a leading Australian researcher in the field. Accessed 16/4/14.

Australasian College of Health Informatics: http://www.achi.org.au/ accessed 16/4/14. The Australasian College of Health Informatics is the professional body for Health Informatics in the Asia–Pacific Region. The credentialed Fellows and Members of the College are national and international experts, thought leaders and trusted advisers in Health Informatics. ACHI sets standards for education and professional practice in Health Informatics, supports initiatives, facilitates collaboration and mentors the community.

Health Informatics Society Australia: Nurse Informatics Australia http://www.hisa.org.au/members/group.aspx?id=85335.

Nursing Informatics Australia (NIA) is the pre-eminent group of nursing informaticians in Australia. This HISA SIG is a good reference point to learn about the developments in Nursing Informatics both nationally and internationally. Over the last decade the health care environment has seen a transformation of work practices and an explosion in the use of information and communication technologies.

http://imia-medinfo.org/ni/welcome accessed16/4/14.

Consistent with the tendencies driven by IMIA, the International Medical Informatics Association, Nursing Informatics Special Interest Group (IMIA NI SIG) updated the definition of nursing informatics emphasising that 'Nursing informatics science and practice integrates nursing, its information and knowledge and their management with information and communication technologies to promote the health of people, families and communities worldwide.'

http://www.amia.org/programs/working-groups/nursing-informatics accessed16/4/14.

Nursing informatics is the 'science and practice (that) integrates nursing, its information and knowledge, with management of information and communication technologies to promote the health of people, families, and communities worldwide.' (IMIA Special Interest Group on Nursing Informatics 2009).

http://www.conno.org.au/members/34-nursing-informatics-australia-nia, accessed 16/4/14.

Nursing Informatics Australia (NIA) is one of a number of special interest groups within the main organisation of the Health Informatics Society Australia (HISA), and is the pre-eminent nursing informatics organisation in Australia.

National e-health Transition Strategy (NEHTA) http://www.nehta.gov.au/our-work/ clinical-terminology/snomed-clinical-terms/educational-resources accessed17/4/14. eHealth brings together the technologies of unique identification, authentication and encryption to provide the foundations and solutions for the safe and secure exchange of healthcare information.

References

Ash, JS, Berg, M & Coiera E 2004, 'Some unintended consequences of information technology in health care: the nature of patient care information system related errors', *J Am Inform Assoc* vol. 11, pp. 104–12.

Australian Government, Department of Health. Welcome to e-health: http://www.ehealth. gov.au/internet/ehealth/publishing.nsf/content/home

Australian Government, Department of Health. Personally Controlled Electronic Health record: http://www.ehealth.gov.au/internet/ehealth/publishing.nsf/content/home

Australian Health Ministers' Conference (AHMC) 2008, *National eHealth strategy*, Victorian Department of Human Services (www.ahmac.gov.au).

Bauer, AM, Thielke, SM, Katon, W. et al 2014, 'Aligning health information technologies with effective service delivery models to improve chronic disease care' *Preventitive Care* (in press)

Boisvert, S 2012, 'Getting to zero: technology. An enterprise look at mHealth', *Journal of Healthcare Risk Management*, vol. 32, no. 2, pp. 44–52.

Brewster, L, Mountain, G, Wessels, B, Kelly, C & Hawley, M 2014, 'Factors affecting front line staff acceptance of telehealth technologies: a mixed-method systematic review', *Journal of Advanced Nursing*, vol. 70, no. 1, pp. 21–33.

Chang, J, Poynton, MR, Gassert, C & Staggers, N 2011, 'Nursing informatics competencies required by nurses in Taiwan', *International Journal of Medical Informatics*, vol. 80, pp. 332–40.

Fairbrother, P, Ure, J, Hanley, J, McCloughan, L, Denvir, M, Sheikh, A, McKinstry, B & the Telescot programme team 2014, 'Telemonitoring for chronic heart failure: the views of patients and healthcare professionals— a qualitative study', *Journal of Clinical* Nursing, vol. 23, no. 1–2, pp. 132–144

Griffiths, F, Cave, J, Boardman, F et al 2012, 'Social networks: the future of healthcare delivery', *Social Science and Medicine*, vol. 75, issue 12, pp. 2233–41.

Handel, MJ 2011, *Explore*, July/August, vol. 7, no.4, pp. 256–61.

Harris, MA, Hood, KK & Mulvaney, SS 2012, 'Pumpers, skypers, surfers and texters: technology to improve the management of diabetes in teenagers', *Diabetes, Obesity and Metabolism*, vol. 14, no. 11, pp. 967–72.

Harvey, MJ & Harvey, MG 2014, 'Privacy and security issues for mobile health platforms', *Journal of the Association for Information Science and Technology*, vol 65. issue 7, pp. 1305–1318.

Hovenga, E 2014, 'The growing specialty of nursing informatics', *NurseClick* August 2013,Australian College of Nursing, pp. 14-16 http://www.acn.edu.au/sites/default/files/publications/nurseclick/acn_nurseclick_august_2013_non-member.pdf accessed 16/4/14

Kabashiki. IR 2013, 'Mobile health means better health care for all', *Journal of Selected Areas in Health Informatics (JSHI)* July, vol. 3(7), pp. 1–13.

Lederman, R, Hanmei, F & Smith S 2014, 'Who can you trust? Credibility assessment in online health forums', *Health Policy and Technology*, 3, 13–25.

Lindley, J & Fernando J 2013, 'Being smart: challenges in the use of mobile applications in clinical settings', *European Journal of ePractice*, no. 21, pp. 4–13.

Moren A, Merete, L & Knudsen, K 2013, 'Nursing informatics: decades of contribution to health informatics', *Health Inform Res*, vol. 19(2), pp. 86–92.

National eHealth Transition Authority 2012, ehealth presentation: http://www.youtube.com/watch?v=JwDTxvkBk-I accessed 17/4/14.

Simpson, R 2011, 'Ethical considerations of nursing informatics', in H Strachan (ed) *Evidence-based practice in nursing informatics*, IGL Global Disseminator of Knowledge, chapter 10.

Strachan, H, Murray, P & Erdley, WS 2011, 'Nursing informatics history and its contributions to nursing knowledge', in H Strachan (ed) *Evidence-based practice in nursing informatics*, IGL Global Disseminator of Knowledge, chapter 7.

Usher, K et al. 2014, 'Australian Health professions student use of social media', *Collegian* Article in Press.

While, A & Dewsbury G 2011, 'Nursing and communication technology (ICT): a discussion of trends and future directions', *International Journal of Nursing Studies*, 48, 1302–10.

Zang, Y, Monsen, KA, Adam, TJ et al. 2011, 'Systematic refinement of health information technology time and motion workflow instrument for inpatient nursing care using a standardized interface terminology', *AMIA Ann Symp Proc* 2011, pp. 1621–9.

14 Lifelong Learning and the Registered Nurse

MARIA FEDORUK

LEARNING OBJECTIVES

After reading this chapter, you will be able to:

- discuss the principles underpinning professional nursing practice
- embed lifelong learning principles into your personal and professional life
- develop a professional portfolio
- develop short-term and long-term career plans.

KEY TERMS

Career planning
Continuing professional development
Curriculum vitae (CV)
Lifelong learning
SWOT analysis

Introduction

The purpose of this chapter is to introduce you to the concept of ongoing professional development for new registered nurses. In preceding chapters in this textbook you will have read about the healthcare system you are about to enter as a registered nurse, and the employment issues facing all health professionals entering the healthcare workforce for the first time (see chapter 7, Australia's healthcare system). There is now an emphasis on measuring performance of individuals against standards as part of the safety and quality imperatives shaping the practices of health professionals (see chapter 11, Safety, quality and the registered nurse). The standards for registered nurses are the Nursing and Midwifery Board of Australia Standards (NMBA 2013). These standards were first published in 2006 but were rebranded in 2013 and are available from http://www.nursingmidwiferyboard.gov.au/Codes-Guidelines-Statements/Codes-Guidelines.aspx#competencystandards.

You will have been introduced to these standards in your undergraduate nursing program, and by now should be familiar with how they underpin professional nursing practice. You will also have noticed that the standards encompass not only the clinical dimensions of nursing practice but the behavioural dimensions.

Therefore, the professional registered nurse is not only clinically competent but also behaves in a professional manner. The professional manner is reflected in dressing appropriately, the interprofessional relationships and interactions with other health professionals, and the relationships developed with patients, their families and carers. Inherent in professional nurse behaviour is treating other people with respect, dignity and cultural awareness. The NMBA (2013) code of conduct for professional nurses should underpin all aspects of your professional practice (http://www.nursingmidwiferyboard.gov.au/Codes-Guidelines-Statements/Codes-Guidelines.aspx#competencystandards; http://www.ahpra.gov.au/Registration/Registration-Process/Standard-Format-for-Curriculum-Vitae.aspx).

Continuing Professional Development

Continuing professional development is mandatory for continuing nurse registration. Continuing professional development is a registration standard approved by the Australian Health Workforce Ministerial Council pursuant to the 2009 *Health Practitioner Regulation National Law Act* (the National Law) and approved from July 1 2010 (NMBA 2013). Continuing professional development for the registered nurse is enshrined in legislation and ignoring this has the potential to compromise your registration to practice.

Lifelong Learning

Linked to continuing professional development is the principle of **lifelong learning**. Learning continues formally and informally throughout your life. Lifelong learning has been identified as an 'imperative for professional nursing and the Institutes of Medicine (IOM) recommend that nurses engage in lifelong learning because it is essential for professional nursing practice' (Davis et al. 2014, p. 441; Krautscheid 2014; Jarvis 2005). Lifelong learning, by definition, extends beyond the completion of the undergraduate program.

Lifelong learning for professional nurses is the continual accumulation of competencies, underpinned by the meshing of knowledge and experience (Jarvis 2005). You will have been introduced to the principles of lifelong learning in your undergraduate nursing program, because lifelong learning is embedded in a university's graduate qualities framework. The graduate qualities may be aspirational but, in marketing terms, they describe a university's product, 'the successful graduate'. You should take the time to read through the graduate qualities of your university and see whether they describe you.

CONTINUING PROFESSIONAL DEVELOPMENT — The methods, by which you as a registered nurse maintain, improve and broaden your knowledge, expertise and competence to continue to develop the professional qualities required of a registered nurse.

LIFELONG LEARNING — The continual accumulation of competencies, complementing knowledge and experience using formal and informal learning methods.

MARIA FEDORUK

Student assessments at universities are designed to align with the university's graduate qualities and the specific course (subject) objectives. Take the time to read through your assessments and note how the assessments have been designed to meet the objectives and lifelong learning graduate quality. Lifelong learning is also linked to the application of knowledge to practice. Nursing is a practice-based discipline whose practitioners use evidence-based knowledge to inform their practice. Developing effective lifelong learning habits will support your career progression into the future because they link with professional standards of nursing practice.

Career Planning

CAREER PLANNING — The systematic approach to planning your career. It includes evaluating strengths and weaknesses; setting goals and objectives, seeking and preparing for career opportunities, and engaging with relevant professional development activities.

Career planning is important for all health professionals, especially registered nurses. The clinical placement may provide you with opportunities to begin your career planning (McKenna et al. 2010). As healthcare systems undergo continual reform processes, cost containment strategies focus on reducing nurse workforce numbers simply because nurses are the largest workgroup in any healthcare organisation. Registered nurses are particularly vulnerable because there is a perceived wisdom that registered nursing work may be done by less qualified and less skilled healthcare workers. This approach to cost containment continues to occur despite solid research evidence showing that the presence of registered numbers is necessary for the delivery of safe, competent nursing care (Blegen et al. 2008; Needleman et al. 2011; Aiken et al. 2012; Aiken et al. 2013).

It is important that you take a strategic approach to planning your career. In your early days as a student nurse you may still not be sure about your future nursing career but you should use your clinical placement experiences to support your career planning.

Each one of you is different, and so your approach to career planning will be different. Most universities have websites devoted to career planning and there are career advisers whom you can contact. It may be appropriate for you to do this, perhaps in your final year of study. The Transition to Professional Practice Program (TPPP) will provide you with opportunities to decide on a clinical career, and you should take advantage of the opportunities presented to you.

Most universities have career advisory services, so you should check your teaching institution's website for links to career planning advice. Some teaching institutions also organise career expos and/or invite speakers from industry to speak to students about future career options. Take every opportunity to obtain as much information as you can.

Whatever your circumstances, career planning is essential, especially in an environment where registered nurse positions are rigorously contested. The career choices and decisions you make will impact not only on you but also on those around you (family, friends and colleagues) and on your nursing practice. It is wise to make the decision that is right for you, because your career is such an important part of your life. You should feel happy and satisfied with your choice of career.

However, you should also allow yourself some flexibility. Career opportunities for nurses may change as technology and demands for health services change, so your career pathway should be developmental. Career opportunities for nurses are expanding and you need to keep your career goals current, because this will enable you to develop and plan your career strategies. Some of you may use the knowledge and competencies you develop as a nurse to move in other career directions at some time in the future. Futurists predict that in the twenty-first century the average person will need to engage in career construction, because careers will be organised differently and job transitions will become more frequent and complex.

SWOT analysis

A strategic approach to career planning begins with a **SWOT analysis**. A SWOT analysis is a simple framework used in project management but which can also be used to assess career opportunities. SWOT stands for strengths, weaknesses, opportunities and threats.

SWOT ANALYSIS —
An acronym
(strengths,
weaknesses,
opportunities and
threats) that describes
a management tool
used for considering
the pros and cons of
a situation, including
career planning.

TABLE 14.1 SWOT ANALYSIS

Strengths	Weaknesses
Opportunities	Threats

This analytic framework can be very helpful in planning your career in nursing, but first you must have a specific career goal in mind. For example, if your goal is to be a nurse practitioner, then by using a SWOT analysis you will be able to identify:

- *your strengths*—competencies and knowledge that you already have but which will have to be further developed to expert status
- *your weaknesses*—areas of your practice which need serious work if you are to achieve your goal. This may include specific courses in the Master of Nurse Practitioner program and working in clinical areas which will enable you to further develop the skills and competencies you will need to achieve your career goal

- *your opportunities*—be alert to opportunities in your workplace that may support your career goals such as conferences that are in your clinical area of interest that will not only enhance your knowledge but also introduce you to nurse experts already working in the area
- *your threats*—an obvious threat may be competition from other registered nurses with the same career goals and aspirations as you, or a hostile environment that does not support professional development.

Having completed your SWOT analysis, it is then time to develop your **curriculum vitae (CV)**.

The Australian Health Practitioner Regulation Agency (AHPRA) and provides a template for a CV (http://www.ahpra.gov.au/Registration/Registration-Process/Standard-Format-for-Curriculum-Vitae.aspx).

It is important that your CV is kept current. A good way of ensuring this is by incorporating your CV into a professional portfolio. A professional portfolio is a collection of documents that show evidence of your competencies, illustrating your expertise—your engagement with continuing professional development activities. The professional portfolio is a record of your professional development as a registered nurse and you may use it to record work-based reflections. Recording work-based reflections may be a useful way to critically appraise and link your clinical experiences and classroom studies.

As a part of nurse registration requirements, the professional portfolio may be audited by the NMBA to ensure your compliance with registration standards, so keeping accurate written records of your nursing experiences is important.

Both the CV and professional portfolio are 'living documents'; that is, as you move through your career, significant achievements are recorded and added. Your CV and professional portfolio may be kept electronically and/or be paper-based. This is important when you decide to apply for promotional positions in the future; the relevant information is in one place.

CURRICULUM VITAE (CV) — A document that summarises your qualifications; work/practice history; clinical skills/competencies and any gaps in your work/practice history.

THEORY TO PRACTICE

The 'bad' patient

During the course of your undergraduate program, you will probably have encountered the stereotypes 'good patient' and 'bad patient'. The 'good patient' is compliant, obeys the nurse's directives, and does not use the call bell often, if at all. The 'bad patient' is always asking for assistance and always ringing the call bell.

You observe an instance of a nurse ignoring the persistent ringing of a call bell. When you ask the nurse allocated to the patient why she does not respond to the patient, you are told 'they're always ringing for something and I'm getting sick of it. If you are so worried, you go and see what they want!'

So you do go and see the patient, who tells you that he is experiencing chest pain and asks for pain relief. You return to your colleague and suggest that it might be appropriate to assess the patient's chest pain and any other symptoms and perhaps call for a medical review. The nurse comments that this patient is a 'wuss', always complaining about something, and she continues to ignore the patient. While you are still discussing the patient, he has a cardiac arrest. He is successfully resuscitated.

Discussion Questions

1. Which competency and registration standards appear to have been breached?
2. How professional was the behaviour of the other nurse on a scale of 1–5, where 1 is very bad and 5 is very good.
3. Where do you sit on this professional continuum?

Critical reflection

Did you write your reflections in your portfolio? Were you prepared to discuss these with colleagues in a tutorial group or workshop?

Applying for a Position

When you first decide to apply for a job, it is useful to do a SWOT (strengths, weaknesses, opportunities and threats) analysis on yourself. Reflecting on your current performance as a registered nurse:

- What are your strengths?
- Which areas of your nursing practice do you believe need further development?
- What are the opportunities available to you in terms of career development? Are these in the area you are currently employed in? Or do you see yourself moving into other areas of nursing practice or even other organisations?
- What are potential threats to you when applying for new positions?

Critical reflection

Use the SWOT analysis framework to begin planning your career. Reflect on your
- strengths
- weaknesses
- opportunities
- threats.

When completing your SWOT analysis, be objective and honest with yourself. During your clinical placements you will have received evaluations which highlighted your strengths and weaknesses—use these to help you. Most of us tend to focus on our weaknesses, but it is also important to focus on our strengths. For example, if in one of your clinical placements your evaluation indicated that one of your strengths was that you were a good communicator, how could you build on this to enhance your communication competencies? A weakness may have been something to do with time management—you had a tendency to be late in completing functions. Reflect on this, and consider what support you would require to improve your time management skills.

Having completed the SWOT analysis on yourself, then consider where you want to work and why. Some of you may be offered employment in the hospitals or healthcare agencies where you spent time on clinical placement or where you have worked as an enrolled nurse (EN) or Assistant in Nursing (AIN). Choose your referees carefully. Referees' comments should enhance and support your CV and the evidence in your professional portfolio.

Where to look for a position

The internet has made job seeking a lot easier: you can search for jobs online and send in your job applications electronically. If you are looking to move to a new healthcare organisation, check their website—the majority of healthcare organisations now list available positions on their websites. Alternatively, go to the Department of Health website and see what positions are available within the public health sector in your state or territory, or in other places around the country. The major papers, especially the weekend papers, list vacancies, and these papers have dedicated employment websites. State and territory departments of health may also list vacancies. Professional nursing journals, career expos and the career advisory service of your university are also good sources for employment opportunities.

There is also the 'cold call' approach, in which you contact the human resources department or the nursing department of the hospital or healthcare agency where you want to work and make enquiries about potential positions. The 'cold call' approach demonstrates initiative, which can be very appealing to employers. You may then be invited to submit a letter of application and your CV and professional portfolio.

The application letter

Your letter of application and professional portfolio are critical, because the decision to interview you will be made on the basis of the information provided in these documents. The application letter should introduce you to the prospective employer, stating your reasons for applying for a position, and outlining why you should be considered for it. It should therefore contain a brief summary of your competencies and knowledge. Try and be succinct with your information: your potential employer and their staff are busy people and do not have the time to read two or three pages. You will expand on your strengths during the interview. The purpose of the application letter is to get you to the interview stage.

The interview

Whatever the format of the interview, you need to be prepared with the correct documentation and evidence of your suitability for the position for which you have applied. For the TPPP, the interview may be with nurse managers or managed centrally by the Department of Health. For more senior positions, it may be a panel interview. If you are being interviewed for a nursing position interstate or overseas, it may be a telephone interview.

Prior to the interview, some organisations will mail you a series of questions to answer. This is a means of checking your literacy levels, your capacity for analysis and your written communication competencies.

Now that you have reached the interview stage, you do not want to compromise your chances of being successful by interviewing badly. Once you know that you are to be interviewed, you should research the organisation by accessing their website—find out what the organisational philosophy is, what the philosophy of the nursing service is and which clinical services are offered. Plan any questions you may want to ask at the interview, because interviews are not one-sided—you will have the opportunity to ask questions of your prospective employer.

For the interview itself:

- Dress appropriately—T-shirts, shorts, thongs, excessive jewellery and heavy makeup are not appropriate. Clothes should be neat, clean and pressed, and should fit you comfortably. If your clothes make you uncomfortable, it will be hard to make a good impression with the interview panel.
- Arrive early—this will give you time to check your appearance and tidy up if necessary. It also gives you time to mentally prepare by doing some relaxation techniques such as deep breathing and going over any documentation you may have brought with you.
- Always try and make eye contact with the person asking the question and then be inclusive of others on the interview panel when responding to questions.
- If your mind suddenly goes blank during a question, ask if you can return to the question later in the interview.
- Try and relax during the interview, although this can be difficult—remember you are at the interview because the organisation wants you.

Taking Care of Yourself

Believe it or not, taking care of yourself is also an important part of your professional development. If you are not fit, healthy and mentally alert, you will not be able to care for your patients in a safe and competent way. As a new registered nurse, change becomes a constant in your life. As a registered nurse, your colleagues and patients hold certain expectations of you, and you may well also place certain expectations on yourself. These factors are coupled with demanding workloads in hospitals and other healthcare facilities resulting from the implementation of efficiency measures and changes to service delivery systems that 'have replaced length of stay with increased patient acuity' (Duchscher & Myrick 2008, p. 191).

Nursing is a stressful occupation, and stress can have an impact on levels of job satisfaction as well, causing psychological and physical ill health (Chang et al. 2006). Some stressors identified by graduate nurses include:

- lacking confidence in your abilities to work as a registered nurse
- a fear of making mistakes because of increased workloads and responsibilities
- having to negotiate new environments and social structures
- learning to work with new staff
- working in a unit that is continually understaffed
- working with unhappy nurses
- not knowing who to go to for help
- being marginalised from other nurses in the clinical unit
- having to demonstrate and apply new knowledge and skills.

As a registered nurse, you have a responsibility to look after yourself in order to be effective as a nurse caring for patients. As a student nurse and as a registered nurse, you should make taking care of yourself a priority, or you may find yourself burning out (Zerwekh & Claborn 2009). Signs of burnout include:

- depression
- feelings of helplessness
- frequent headaches and gastrointestinal disturbances
- insomnia
- being continually negative—a 'glass half empty' person
- cynicism
- always being tired
- weight fluctuations
- self-criticism—the 'I'm no good/can't do anything right' syndrome (Zerwekh & Claborn 2009, p. 35).

Do any of these signs apply to you? If they do, then you should take action immediately, using the strategies listed below.

Learning to care for yourself means developing self-awareness of your feelings and knowing how to deal with them. Nurses who have good emotional health are able to deal with their emotions appropriately without embarrassing themselves or others. You need to express your feelings, especially negative feelings, to avoid them becoming internalised to such an extent that you begin to develop some of the symptoms listed above.

THEORY TO PRACTICE

You and your friend Jane are out on your final clinical placement. As this is your final placement, both you and Jane want to make a good impression on the registered nurses who are working with you. For the first two weeks, you and Jane work well with other members of the multidisciplinary team; their feedback is positive, and you are hopeful that your evaluation from this venue will be positive and you will be able to use this to support your application for a TPPP position in this very same venue.

In week 3 of the placement, you notice a change in Jane. She has become withdrawn, does not engage with other team members and has made some errors when delivering care to her allocated patients. The Nurse Unit Manager asks you if you know what is causing Jane to behave in this way.

Discussion Questions

1. Do you approach Jane directly and ask her what is bothering her?
2. Do you ask Jane to speak with the Nurse Unit Manager?
3. Do you speak with the university lecturer and ask them to speak with Jane?
4. Is it important that Jane's issues are managed correctly and within policy boundaries?
5. Is Jane placing herself at risk by not acknowledging her behaviour and seeking help?
6. Which registration standard is Jane breaching?

Self-care strategies

Here are some strategies to help you avoid or deal with stress in the life of a registered nurse:

- Manage your physical environment—ensure that it is hazard-free, safe and tidy.
- Manage your time effectively. Plan and prioritise. Do not buy into the myth of the perfect nurse.
- Deal with procrastination. Think about the potential consequences of not doing something, compared to doing something.

- Learn to delegate. You are not 'super nurse'.
- Manage your personal and professional goals through a professional portfolio.
- Engage in physical exercise. Many healthcare organisations now have gyms on site that offer subsidised membership to staff.
- Walk for at least 20 minutes a day.
- Take stretch breaks while at work.
- Learn to laugh, and laugh frequently.
- Remember to have fun. Take up a relaxing hobby such as doing puzzles or Sudoku.

There is a great deal of information available for you to discover what sort of activities help you keep healthy.

You may feel that between your home and work commitments you do not have time to do all this. You need to *make* the time unless you want to become a statistic. To paraphrase Henry Thoreau: 'We are all busy but what are we busy about?' How can you deliver good health messages to patients when you are obviously not heeding your own advice?

SUMMARY

This chapter has focused on professional development in nursing and how this is determined by the NMBA competence framework. The requirements for continuing registration as a registered nurse and midwife include using an evidence-based professional portfolio. Nurse and midwives are expected to take a strategic approach to managing their careers and assume responsibility for their professional development. Even though there is a reported nursing workforce shortage, healthcare organisations are still looking for nurses who are safe, competent, professional practitioners and who will fit in and work with their organisational philosophy and mission statements.

An integral part of your professional development is maintaining your own physical and mental well-being. Nursing is a stressful occupation, with competing demands on nurses wherever nurses work. Nursing literature is now discussing the adverse effects on new graduates of workload stress at the national and international levels. The factors that contribute to workload stress in nurses are universal—you are not alone in experiencing the workload stress phenomenon.

As a graduate nurse, you have the added stressors of entering a new work environment in a new role that brings with it different expectations and responsibilities. The section on taking care of yourself in this chapter outlines the risks and also provides strategies for minimising the effects of workload stress. There are many strategies available to you: the most important thing is to use the one that works for you.

Discussion questions

1. What are three 'take home' messages for you from this chapter?
2. How important is career management and planning to you?
3. In a group, discuss you career development plans. You could look at where you hope to be in three years' time. What will you need to do to achieve your career goals?
4. Where will you go to access resources to support your career development? How will understanding the transition process help you achieve your career goals?
5. What are some of the strategies you use to take care of yourself?

Further Reading

Registration standards: http://www.nursingmidwiferyboard.gov.au/Registration-Standards.aspx.

Codes, guidelines: http://www.nursingmidwiferyboard.gov.au/Codes-Guidelines-Statements/Codes-Guidelines.aspx.

Social Media Policy: http://www.nursingmidwiferyboard.gov.au/Codes-Guidelines-Statements/Codes-Guidelines/Social-media-policy.aspx.

Mid-Staffordshire NHS Public Inquiry 2010: http://www.midstaffspublicinquiry.com/report

Marquis, BL & Huston CJ 2014, 'Career development: From new graduate to retirement', in Marquis & Huston, *Leadership roles and management functions in nursing*, Wolters Kluwer/Lippincottt Williams & Wilkins, 8th edn. pp. 228–51.

Useful websites

Nursing and Midwifery Board of Australia: http://www.nursingmidwiferyboard.gov.au/.
Australian Health Practitioner Regulation Agency: http://www.ahpra.gov.au/.
Department of Health-Employment: http://www.health.gov.au/internet/main/publishing.nsf/Content/Capability+Map.
SA Health Careers: http://www.sahealthcareers.com.au/story/.

References

Aiken, LH, Sloane, DM, Bruyneel, L, Van den Heede, K, Sermeus W for the RN4 CAST Consortium 2013, 'Nurses' report of working conditions and hospital quality of care in 12 countries in Europe', *International Journal of Nursing Studies*, vol. 50, pp. 143–53.

Aiken, LH, Sermeus, W, Van den Heede, K, Sloane, DM, Busse, R et al. 2012, 'Patient safety, satisfaction and quality of hospital care: cross sectional surveys of nurses and patients in 12 countries in Europe and the United States', *BMJ* 344: e 1717, pp. 1–14.

Blegen, M, Vaughn T & Vojir C 2008, 'Nurse staffing levels: impact of organizational characteristics and registered nurse supply', *Health Services Research*, vol. 43 (pt 1), pp. 154–73.

Chang, EM, Daly, JW, Hancock, KM et al. 2006, 'The relationship among workplace stressors, coping methods, demographic characteristics and health: Australian nurses', *Journal of Professional Nursing*, vol. 22, issue 1, pp. 30–38.

Davis, L, Taylor, H & Reyes, H 2014, 'Lifelong learning in nursing: a Delphi study', *Nurse Education Today*, vol. 34, pp. 441–43.

Duchscher, JEB & Myrick, F 2008, 'The prevailing winds of oppression: understanding the new graduate experience in acute care,' *Nursing Forum*, vol. 43, no. 4, pp. 191–8.

Dwyer, J & Hopwood, N 2013, *Management strategies and skills*, McGraw-Hill, Australia.

Goleman, D 2005, *Emotional intelligence*, Bantam Books, New York.

Jarvis, P 2005, 'Lifelong education and its relevance to nursing' *Nurse Education Today*, vol. 25, pp. 655–60.

Krautscheid, LC, 2014, Defining professional nursing accountability: a literature review. *Journal of Professional Nursing*, vol. 30, no. 1 (January/February), pp. 43–7.

Marquis, BL & Huston, CJ 2012, *Leadership roles and management functions in nursing*, 7th edn, Wolters Kluwer/Lippincott Williams & Wilkins, Philadelphia.

McKenna, L, Mc Call, L & Wray, N 2010, 'Clinical placements and nursing students' career planning: a qualitative exploration', *International Journal of Nursing Practice*, vol. 16, pp. 176–82.

Needleman, J, Buerhaus, P, Pankrantz, VS, Leibson CL, Stevens SR & Harris M 2011, Nurse staffing and inpatient hospital mortality. *New England Journal Medicine*, vol. 364 (11) pp. 1037–45.

Zerwekh, J & Claborn JC 2009 *Nursing today: Transitions and trends*, 6th edn, Saunders Elsevier, St. Louis MI.

Glossary

Accreditation

A process of evaluating and measuring organisational performance (clinical and non-clinical) against national standards.

Australian Commission on Safety and Quality in Healthcare

A government agency that leads and coordinates national improvements in safety and quality across Australia.

Belongingness

The socialisation process an individual goes through to become a member of a new group.

Career planning

The systematic approach to planning your career. It includes evaluating strengths and weaknesses; setting goals and objectives, seeking and preparing for career opportunities, and engaging with relevant professional development activities.

Civil law

Enables individuals, singly and collectively to resolve disputes and differences of a personal and property nature that arise between members of a community and which are unable to be resolved by the parties involved (Staunton & Chiarella, 2013, p. 9).

Clinical assessment

An evaluation of a person's state of health based upon the person's medical history, physical examination, and results of associated laboratory tests.

Clinical governance

A system through which healthcare organisations are accountable for continuously improving the quality of their services and safeguarding standards of care.

Clinical leadership

Enables peers to act and enable clinical performance, to improve clinical practice and for nurses it is about improving nursing practice.

Clinical placement

A period of time spent in a health setting where the student has an opportunity to integrate knowledge and practical skills with the goal of meeting specific clinical objectives relevant to a particular course.

Common law

Consists of cases decided by the courts using established common-law principles (Staunton & Chiarella 2013, p. 5).

Communication

The exchange of words, ideas, information through speech, writing, behaviours, facial expressions, tone of voice. Communication can occur at a number of levels but the two most common levels are verbal and non-verbal (Marquis Huston 2012).

Competencies

Capabilities or abilities that include both intent and action that link directly to how well a person performs completing tasks.

Competencies

The bringing together of a range of general attributes, such as knowledge, skills and behaviours, to nursing practice.

Competency standards

The national competency standards for the registered nurse are the core competency standards by which your performance is assessed to obtain and retain your registration as a registered nurse in Australia.

Consent to treatment

This is covered by an area of 'civil law relating to a trio of civil wrongs or torts concerned with 'trespass to the person' (Staunton & Chiarella 2013, p. 137).

Continuing professional development

The methods, by which you as a registered nurse maintain, improve and broaden your knowledge, expertise and competence to continue to develop the professional qualities required of a registered nurse.

Contract of employment

The basis of a health professional's relationship with an employer is that of contract where the employer has the power to direct the manner in which an employee performs work (McIlwraith & Madden 2014, p. 349).

Criminal law

Rules of expected behaviours governing people's conduct in the community and backed by sanctions of punishment in relation to other people and their property (Staunton & Chiarella 2013, p. 8).

Critical appraisal

The 'process of systematically examining research evidence to assess its validity, results and relevance before using it to inform a decision' (Hill & Spittlehouse 2003).

Critical thinking

Complex thinking patterns that examine situations in terms of context and content. Critical thinkers also anticipate the consequences of decision-making.

Cross-cultural communication

A symbolic exchange process whereby individuals from two (or more) different cultural communities negotiate shared meanings in an interactive situation.

Culturally and linguistically diverse (CALD) background

A person who differs from the mainstream culture according to religion and spirituality, racial background and ethnicity, as well as language.

Culture

A learned, patterned behavioural response acquired over time that includes implicit and explicit beliefs, attitudes, values, customs, norms, taboos, arts, and lifeways accepted by a community of individuals.

Curriculum vitae (CV)

A document that summarises your qualifications; work/practice history; clinical skills/competencies and any gaps in your work/practice history.

eHealth

The combined use of communication and information technology in the healthcare sector to deliver the right information to the right person at the right time in a secure electronic environment, to ensure the optimal delivery of safe, quality care to patients. eHealth is the infrastructure that supports information exchange between all healthcare professionals and patients.

Emotional intelligence

Having self-awareness, social awareness, able to manage relationships and able to manage self.

End-of-grant knowledge translation plan

The researcher develops and implements a plan for disseminating findings that includes traditional dissemination activities such as publications in peer-reviewed journals and conference presentations, and additional modes of dissemination.

Ethics

Refers to the various ways of thinking and understanding how to live a moral life.

Evidence-based practice (EBP)

The use of current, best clinical evidence in making patient care decisions, and such evidence typically comes from published research conducted by nurses and other healthcare professionals.

Evidence–practice gap

The degree to which health services for individuals and populations increase the likelihood of desired health outcomes and are consistent with current professional knowledge.

Experiential learning

Making meaning from direct experience to build knowledge; e.g. the knowledge acquired during clinical placement.

Fitting in

An important feature of becoming a registered nurse.

Followership

The process of following leaders. Leadership and followership are interdependent.

Functional flexibility

Role substitution such as replacing registered and/or enrolled nurses with less skilled healthcare workers, such as nurse assistants.

Health literacy

The knowledge and skills required to understand and use information relating to health issues.

Horizontal violence

Antisocial behaviours between members of the same profession where one member(s) bullies another.

Hospital error

Errors that occur in treatment of a patient during an episode of care while in hospital.

Infection control

Actions taken to prevent nosocomial or healthcare-associated infection.

Information management

The collection and analysis of patient-related information by health professionals to plan and provide care and services to patients.

Information systems

The software and hardware used by a healthcare organisation to communicate and record details of activities related to patient care.

Integrated knowledge translation plan

A plan in which potential users of the research knowledge are involved in the entire research process; that is, those who generate research knowledge and those who might use it (end users) work together to shape the research project within a collaborative relationship that is built on trust and cooperation.

Interprofessional collaboration

An 'interprofessional process for communication and decision-making that enables the separate and shared knowledge and skills of care providers to synergistically influence the client/patient care provided' (Way et al. 2000, p. 3).

Interprofessional conflict

Conflicts that occur between members of different health professions.

Interprofessional education

'IPE occurs when two or more professions learn with, from and about each other to improve collaboration and the quality of care' The Centre for the Advancement of Interprofessional Education (CAIPE 2002).

Interprofessional practice

'IPP occurs when all members of the health service delivery team participate in the team's activities and rely on one another to accomplish common goals and improve health care delivery, thus improving patient's quality experience' (AIPPEN).

Intraprofessional conflict

Conflicts that occur between members of the same profession.

Knowledge translation (KT)

The process of moving evidence into practice.

Knowledge-to-action

The translation of research knowledge into clinical practice.

Leadership

Seeing what is in the present, seeing what needs to be done and closing the gap (adapted from G Cummins).

Lifelong learning

The continual accumulation of competencies, complementing knowledge and experience using formal and informal learning methods.

Management

A series of processes comprising assessing, planning, directing, controlling and evaluating to achieve goals. For nurses, management achieves patient goals and outcomes.

mHealth

Healthcare services that are or accessed by mobile devices such as mobile phones, smartphones, laptops and tablets to collect, retrieve and/or deliver health information.

National Healthcare Agreement (NHA)

The National Healthcare Agreement (NHA) defines the goals of the health system. It specifies the roles and responsibilities of the Commonwealth and State governments in improving health outcomes for Australians and ensuring sustainability of the health system. The seven objectives of the National Healthcare Agreements are prevention; primary and community health; hospital and related care; aged care; patient experience; social inclusion and indigenous health and sustainability (CoAG, 2014).

National Safety and Quality Health Service Standards

These standards drive the implementation of safety and quality systems to improve the quality of health care in Australia. The NSQHSS were developed by the ACQSHC.

Numerical flexibility

Attained through practices where nurses' working time is adjusted by asking or requiring part-time/full-time staff to work overtime and/or take time off due to fluctuating patient occupancy levels.

Nursing informatics

Science and practice integrates nursing, its information and knowledge and their management with information and communication technologies to promote the health of people, families and communities worldwide (Hovenga 2013, p. 14).

Nursing research

Scientific inquiry (**qualitative** and **quantitative**) designed to develop knowledge about health and well-being. It is essential for the nursing profession to strengthen its research culture and support evidence-based nursing practice, to optimise the health and well-being of people and society.

Paradigm

A world view that is based on a set of values and philosophical assumptions that are shared by a particular academic community and that guide their approach to research.

Preceptorship

The practice of a student/graduate nurse working with an RN in the practice setting to increase the knowledge and skills application of the student/graduate nurse.

Professional boundaries

Limits which protect the space between the professional's power and the client's vulnerability.

Professional skills escalation

The expectations of people's performance in their jobs. Organisations are demanding greater skills, flexibility and performance of their staff during the time they are at work. This is also referred to as 'work intensification'.

Quality nursing practice

Nursing practice that is competency-based on national standards, where patient outcomes exceed expectations. Data derived from research is used to inform nurses' practice.

Quality of care

The degree to which health services for individuals and populations increase the likelihood of desired health outcomes and are consistent with current professional knowledge.

Registration standards

Registration standards define the requirements that applicants, registrants or students need to meet in order to be registered.

Registration

Occurs once a student nurse completes an accredited undergraduate program, meeting the registration standards requirements from the NMBA.

Regulation

Rules, guidelines and directives that are enforceable through the appropriate laws.

Research

A systematic process used to confirm and refine existing knowledge and to build new knowledge both inductively and deductively.

Risk

The chance or possibility of an event occurring that will have a negative outcome.

Risk management

A program designed to identify, minimise and avoid risks to patients, staff, volunteers, visitors and all people who come into a healthcare organisation.

Safe nursing practice

Nursing practice that is delivered as per standards-based clinical protocols and does not harm the patient.

Skills

Tasks that do not have to be integrated with knowledge and behaviours.

Socialisation

The process of learning behaviours which are acceptable to members of established groups.

Standard

An accepted or approved example of something against which judgments or measurements can be made. A level of quality and/or excellence.

Statutory law

Consists of laws created by Parliament and embodied in documents known as Acts of Parliament, commonly referred to as 'legislation' (Staunton & Chiarella 2013, p. 5).

SWOT analysis

An acronym (strengths, weaknesses, opportunities and threats) that describes a management tool used for considering the pros and cons of a situation, including career planning.

Time management

Organising and prioritising workloads within the time available.

Transcultural nursing

A field of nursing in which the nurse interacts with clients in intercultural encounters, identifies care needs and delivers care that is culturally congruent for the clients.

Transformational leadership

A participative style of leadership that motivates others to achieve goals beyond expectations.

Transition to Professional Practice Program (TPPP)

A 12-month employment opportunity with scheduled professional learning activities and experiences that supports and enables the graduate nurse to adapt to the RN role.

Transition

The changes that occur over a period of time as individuals change from one state to another.

Work—life balance

The balance between work and personal life.

Workplace Health and Safety (WHS)

Nurses need to be aware of the policies and procedures relating to safe practice in their organisations, including the responsibilities of their employer, as well as their responsibilities as an employee under the Workplace Health and Safety (WHS) legislation in their state or territory.

Index